AF439740

IMAGES of TECHNOLOGY

a pictorial dictionary of modern engineering research

edited by
Institute of Industrial Science
University of Tokyo

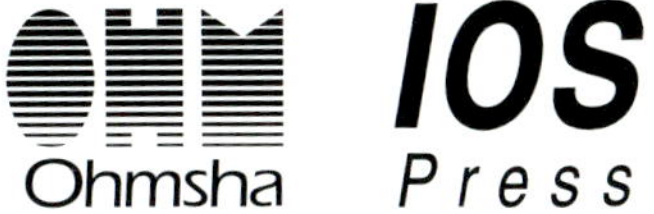

Ohmsha   IOS Press

IMAGES of TECHNOLOGY
          a pictorial dictionary of modern engineering research
Edited by   Institute of Industrial Science, University of Tokyo

Editorial Committee:
Editor - in - Chief   TACHIBANA, Hideki
Head Editor   MAGARIBUCHI, Hidekuni
Editorial Members   ASHIHARA, Satoshi   KOMATSU, Kunitoshi   MIZOBE, Yasushi   SAKAMOTO, Shinichi   SAGA, Tetsuo
                    SEZAKI, Kaoru   TANI, Yasuhiro   WATANABE, Yasuhiro   YOSHIKAWA, Nobuhiro

ISBN 4-274-90323-0 (Ohmsha, Ltd.)
ISBN 1-58603-025-6 (IOS Press)

Publisher:
Ohmsha, Ltd.
3-1 Kanda Nishiki-cho, Chiyoda-ku, Tokyo 101-8460, Japan
fax: +81 3 3293 2824   e-mail: shuppan@ohmsha.co.jp

Distributed in:
Japan by
Ohmsha, Ltd.
3-1 Kanda Nishiki-cho, Chiyoda-ku, Tokyo 101-8460, Japan
fax: +81 3 3233 2426
e-mail: hanbaibu@ohmsha.co.jp

USA and *Canada* by
IOS Press, Inc.
5795-G Burke Center Parkway, Burke, VA 22015, U.S.A.
fax: +1 703 323 3668
e-mail: iosbooks@iospress.com

UK and *Ireland* by
IOS Press
73 Lime Walk, Headington, Oxford, OX3 7AD, England
fax: +44 1865 75 0079

Germany by
IOS Press/Lavis Marketing
Spandauer Strasse 2, D-10178 Berlin, Germany
fax: +49 30 242 3113

Europe and *the rest of the world* by
IOS Press
Van Diemenstraat 94, 1013 CN Amsterdam, Netherlands
fax: +31 20 620 3419
e-mail: order@iospress.nl

Far East jointly by
Ohmsha, Ltd. and IOS Press

preface

The term 'engineering' encompasses quite an extensive overall picture. Until very recently it meant a learning field where the purpose was to make things. It has, in the ongoing effort to make better quality things for people at lower cost, given us roads, buildings, automobiles, an infinite variety of machines, computers, semiconductors, fabrics, chemicals, and countless other things. And further developments and improvements are still being made in each of the sub-fields of engineering—electric devices, machinery, construction and so on.

These things engineering has given us we more or less take for granted today. We consider them an intricate part of the complex world we live in, and sometimes it appears as if we can hardly improve on them, that virtually all of the problems associated with them have been solved.

Against this background the question arises: Where does engineering go from here? This book attempts to answer this question. In doing so, it delves into accomplishments that go beyond the concept of 'fields' in engineering, and combines a number of these to create new fields. And these new fields then bring forth still newer fusions.

Engineering has evolved from a science that merely creates things into one that creates value, solves problems that society faces, and creates things for those purposes. During this time, Institute of Industrial Science, University of Tokyo (I.I.S.) has evolved and continues to evolve in the same way, building on the activities it has engaged in during the past 50 years.

June 1999

Masao Sakauchi
Director General
Institute of Industrial Science
University of Tokyo

contents

discovery

invention

epilogue ·········· 117

book design: Tsuyoshi Aruga

prologue

"Making things" : Something we all do

Japan-bound flights from Europe, after leaving the continent's northern cities in their wake, inevitably must transverse the vast wilderness of Siberia. As they head for the polar ice cap, night flights race through the crisp, clear air that supports them over the barren, untamed land below, gliding through the night sky like some kind of slow-moving shooting star.

One night when I was a passenger on such a flight, while most everyone else was fast asleep, I was gazing out the window at the dark Siberian tundra below. The muted hum of the engines in the Arctic night was in sharp contrast to the ear-splitting roar they had disgorged during takeoff. In this serene silence, the dark land under the midnight sun was drifting backwards as if it was being slowly rolled up—it was like a scene in a hazy dream under a slight fever.

And then I suddenly saw a light flickering on the dark ground below—the light from somebody's house. And it brought home to me a renewed realization that even in such an inhospitable and unyielding environment as Siberia, people will find a way to make a living for themselves. Yet here I am way up in the air, thinking of people's lives down below, while people down there don't even imagine such thoughts are flying over their heads.

On this particular flight, which I had boarded at Paris, I was on my way home from a fact-finding trip to Africa. Unlike the Siberian habitants below me, the people I had been with in Africa the day before had no lights in their homes at all. This in no way means that they were backward or uncivilized, however. When they saw the car we drove to their village, they did not fear it as some sort of great metal beast. Nor did they look at the photo I took of their chief as the devil's work; they were merely excited and happy at seeing it. They instinctively realized that there was some sort of mechanism which enables cars and cameras to do the things they do. They are not able to explain the mechanism of these things in detail, but neither can we.

Using the same kind of logic, they adapt to the climate they live in. They farm and raise livestock, make houses of sun-dried clay, build raised-floor storehouses to guard stores against flooding. They ferment spirits and offer them to visitors who come to them in cars and airplanes. They take money in exchange for goods, build a complex family structure, raise their children in their own way. In doing all of these things, they construct their own version of a full-fledged society.

In a very real sense, then, there is little if any difference between people who ride in cars and airplanes and people who live in homes without lights. Both the village and lifestyle made by one group of people, and the modern passenger planes made by another, illustrate the universal drive of people to create and build.

These thoughts passed through my mind as I gazed at that single light flickering on the dark earth below. It is to my regret that I have never had a chance to visit any persons living in Siberia. However, I have no doubt that when those people down there see a plane passing overhead, they can as human beings identify themselves with those who created that plane. At a very primitive level, we share the concept of "making," going beyond the need to communicate and interact.

*   *   *

Welcome to the world of engineering! If I could, I would be interested to hear what your own image is of making things. My view is that the propensity to make things is one of the most important qualities human beings possess. People have been making things since the dawn of history, and in fact, I think you could even say that the propensity to make things is one of the things that makes us human. In this book, I would like to discuss the advanced climate for making things that has created the world we know today.

These days, just about everything we see is a product of human imagination. Naturally enough in modern cities, but even in the villages of Africa and the dwellings in Siberia, the world is littered with things human beings have made. People have really made their mark on the world through the scope, variety, diversity, and environmental effect of the things they create—all as a result of our unique thought process.

This is a critical point in the field of engineering. In the creative process, people go beyond theoretical limits and use their senses and desires without reasoning everything out. Thus, the making of things quite literally involves using one's imagination. We all possess transcendental sense; as a result our objective in making something is at times simply to make something.

Admonition, however, has from the dawn of history stood in counterpoint to our inclinations and desires. The Bible's Old Testament tells the story of the Tower of Babel (Genesis, Chap. 11), and there is the Hindu god Shiva who destroys to create. Today, however, it appears that the Tower of Babel, which God purportedly destroyed, has changed its form time and again and is continuing to be built today.

And our reward for building the tower is appearing right before our eyes throughout society. Diseases spread through human contact, proliferating weapons of mass destruction, wars, pollution, traffic accidents, depletion of natural resources, global warming, the population boom, spreading slums in our cities—these, too, are things man has created through his own inclinations and desires. It is fair to say that short-sighted creativity, however well-intentioned, can bring disaster upon society.

In the Tower of Babel story, the language of the people becomes confused at the will of God, making it impossible for them to communicate and build cities. These misfortunes too are an integral part of society, but they do much to impede communication and promote misunderstanding. In this sense, it looks as if even today our ability to create things is restricted by the punishments God metes out. In any event, the notion that creating things always brings merit and value to society cannot stand unquestioned in today's complex world.

This being the situation, then, what approach should be taken for the engineering field as a study topic? After all, the object in engineering is to make things—specifically, for people to make things. The first step in evaluating what modern engineering should be is to examine its object and objectives from a broader perspective.

Targets——substance and phenomenon

The traditional targets of engineering have been physical, visible things (i.e., substance). In modern engineering, however, targets also include abstract things without physical substance (i.e., phenomenon). Examples of substance/phenomenon combinations are 'material/flow, wave, vibration', 'hardware/software', 'chemicals/chemical reactions', 'cities, buildings/livelihood', and 'production/design'

Objectives——discovery and invention

In contrast, objectives can be broken down into making things that did not previously exist (invention), and finding things that existed but were not known (discovery).

In making things, the making itself is the actual objective. But in the making process, it is absolutely necessary to ascertain the nature or properties of what is being made. In the same way science as a whole makes an objective of ascertaining the nature of phenomena. In the engineering field, one objective is to discover new phenomena and use them to create new substance.

'New Engineering' and the organization of this book

In fields of learning today, much is made of the need to reconstruct the learning systems established through the use of modern rationalism. For example, traditional learning to learn/make the things one encounters in life encompasses many fields— physics, medicine, engineering, agriculture, philosophy, psychology, sociology. From this viewpoint, it is not an exaggeration to say that the exact same conditions are involved in 'environment', 'society' and so on—the essential issues the times have brought into the field of learning.

The learning systems that classification and fractionalizing have self-completed are doing a great deal to help us further our knowledge in all fields. However, it cannot be doubted that the deepening and heightening of knowledge in these fields—the so-called 'vertical axis' development—is bringing about the imperfections in what should be the 'horizontal axis'—'the complicated, mutually related systems of nature and society'.

To modern engineering, it is only natural that the viewpoint of this 'horizontal axis' should be of extreme importance. When this viewpoint is obtained, engineering will have evolved into a completely new field of learning.

In this book, I have tried to provide an overall perspective of the engineering world by emphasizing the larger meaning of 'object' and 'objective' in this field, without delving into the field's traditional structure.

The chapter on 'substance' and 'phenomena' focuses on the 'object' pursued in engineering as the main point, where 'objective' is the focus in the chapter on 'discovery' and 'invention'.

The thrust of the book is on the four combinations that can be made from the 'object' and 'objective' elements. But each area of research has its own multifaceted background, and it is not enough to rely on such a simple classification. Classification can only be simplified if people revise the very way they view the idea of research. In modern learning, then, it is most important to have an open mind with respect to the position of research in the overall scheme of things.

I.I.S. in society: a 50-year history

The illustrations in this book depict recent research results obtained by Institute of Industrial Science, University of Tokyo (I.I.S.). I.I.S. was founded as an engineering institute at the University of Tokyo in the immediate post-war era, in June of 1949. Today it has become one of the world's top research institutes, both in terms of size and research quality, with over 100 separate labs covering virtually the entire engineering spectrum. As an independent organization, it is recognized as a leader in the engineering field both within and outside Japan.

Engineering has a strong presence in today's society. I.I.S.'s location, at the very center of a modern major metropolis, has enabled its personnel to become acutely aware of the needs and demands of the society of which it is a part. In a way, its 50-year history closely reflects that of society during that period.

Every month since I.I.S. was founded, it has issued a publication 'Seisan-Kenkyu' containing articles on the Institute's research work. The publication's cover hints at the role that I.I.S. has played in society for the past 50 years. The 'history' chapter in this book, written as a promenade linking 'targets (the 'substance', 'phenomenon' chapter) with 'objectives' (the 'discovery', 'invention' chapter), hopefully will offer the reader a further glimpse into this role.

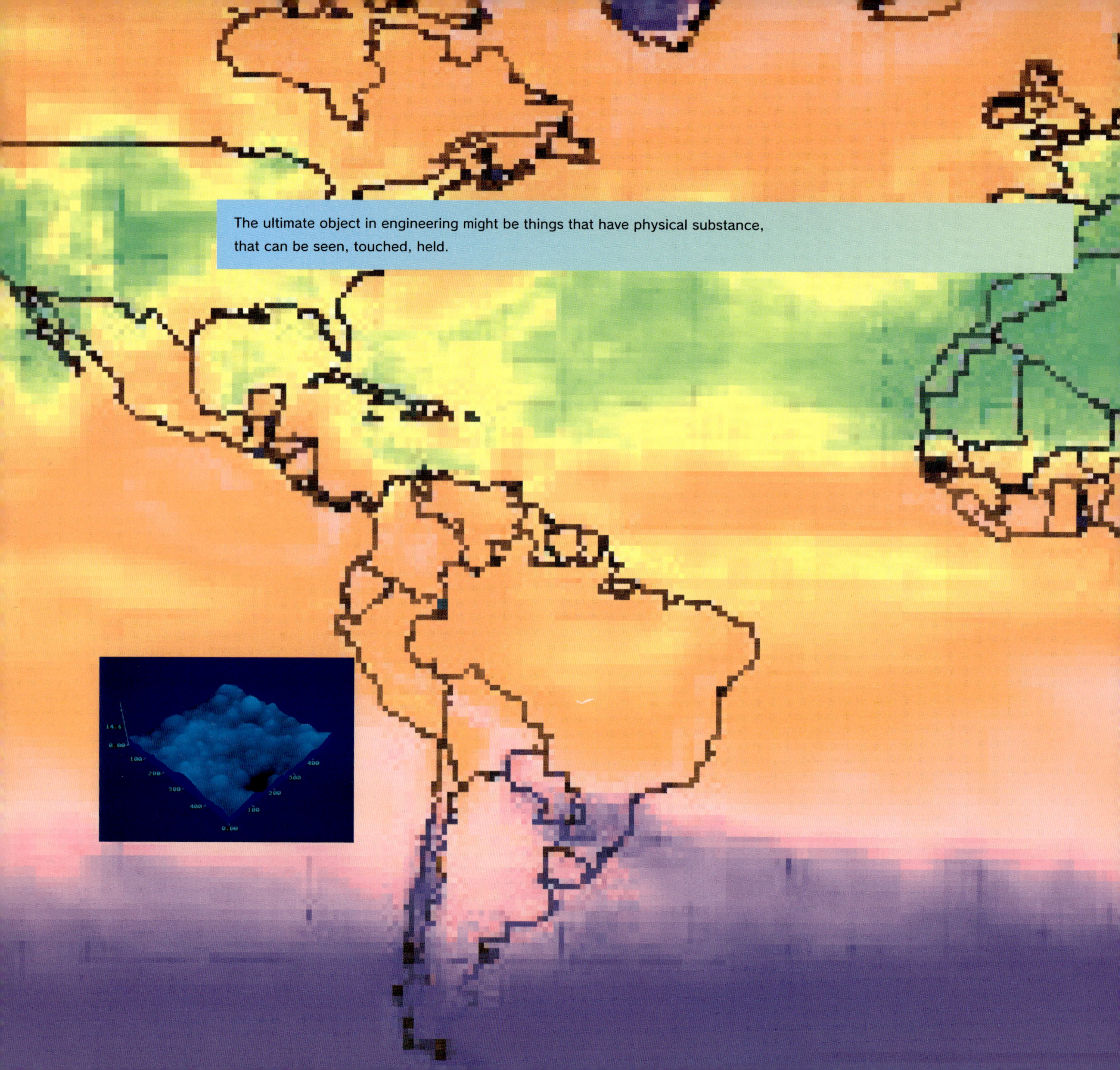
The ultimate object in engineering might be things that have physical substance,
that can be seen, touched, held.

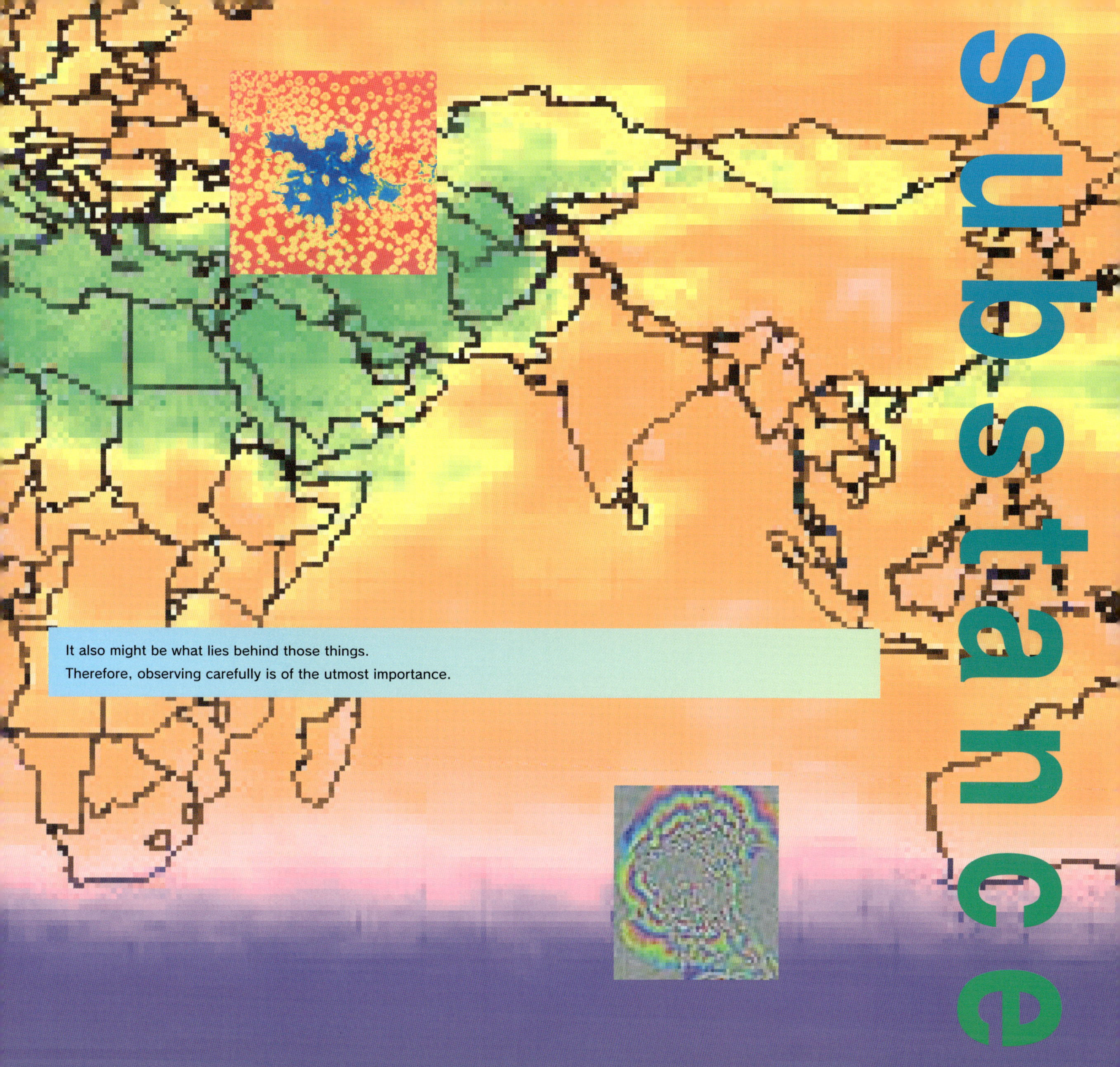

It also might be what lies behind those things.
Therefore, observing carefully is of the utmost importance.
substance

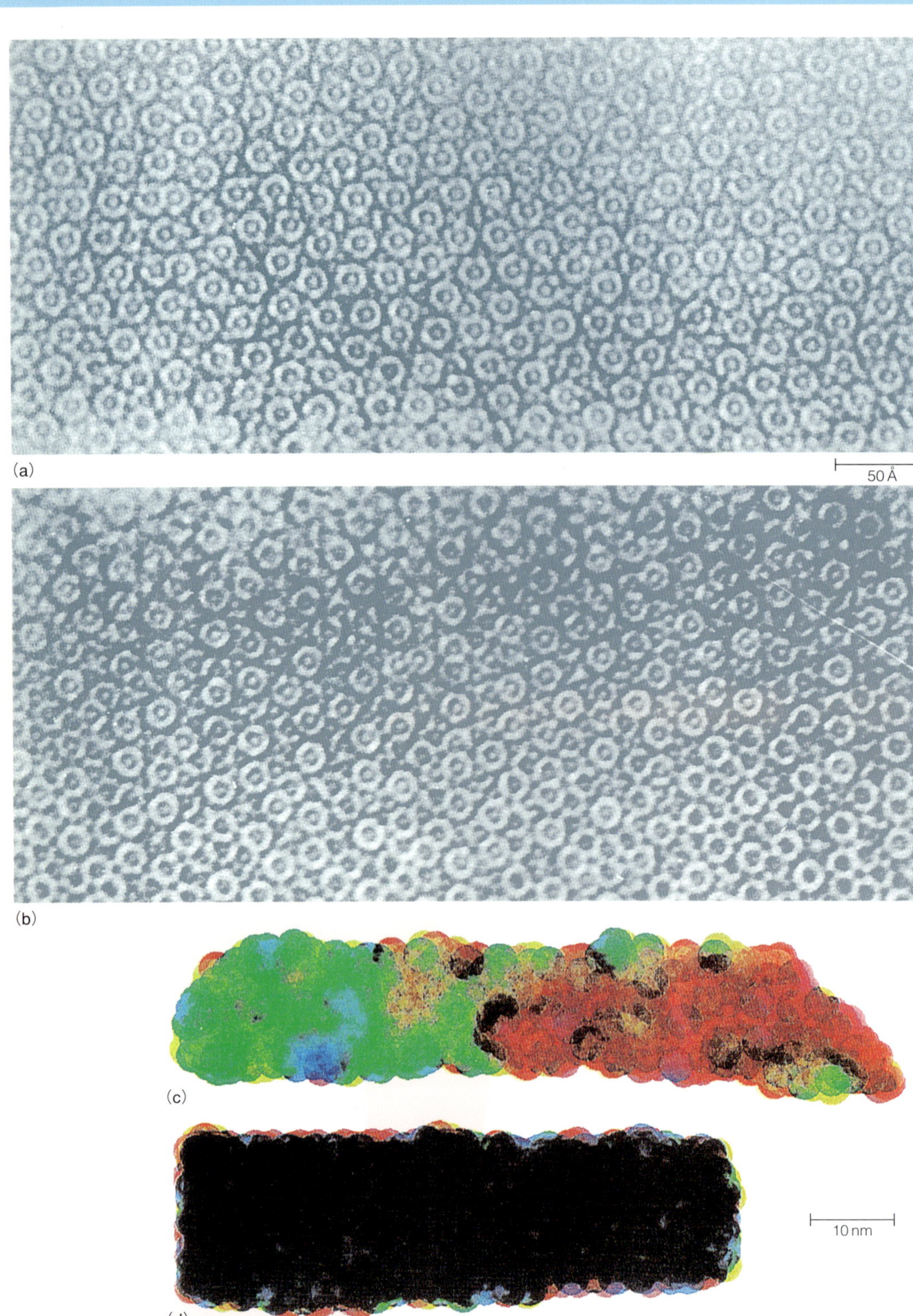

TEM of order-disorder transformation in quasicrystal

The material named quasicrystal, which possesses a crystallographically-forbidden rotational symmetry, has attracted much attention. Fig. (a) and (b) show ordered and disordered states of a quasicrystal observed by high-resolution Transmission Electron Microscopy (TEM) with an atomic resolution of $1 \sim 2$ Å. In fig. (c) and (d), they are image-processed, where the brightness and type of colors indicate the degree of order and type of variant respectively. An atomic rearrangement has been shown to be responsible for the order-disorder transformation.

Every material consists of atoms, which can be as small as one-billionth of a meter. Thanks to the development of various kinds of microscopes, we observe and control an arrangement of atoms with atom-size precision.

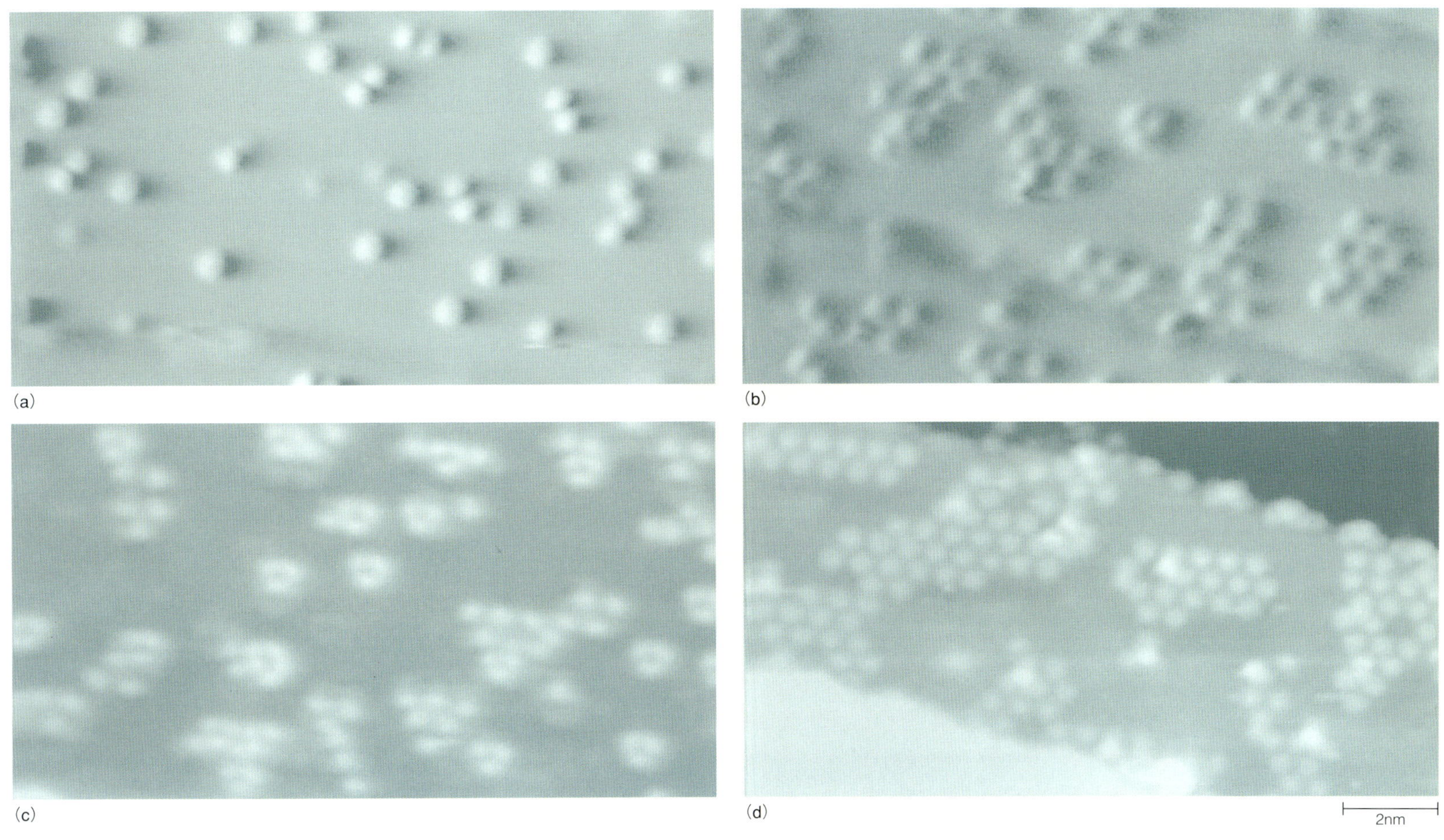

STM images of NO molecules

Scanning Tunneling Microscope (STM) images of nitric oxide molecules adsorbed on a Pt surface obtained at 10 K (fig. (a), (b)) and 70 K (fig.(c), (d)). White circles denote individual molecules. The molecules are isolated from each other at low molecular densities (fig. (a), (c)), while the molecules are arranged in a regular pattern at high densities (fig. (b), (d)).

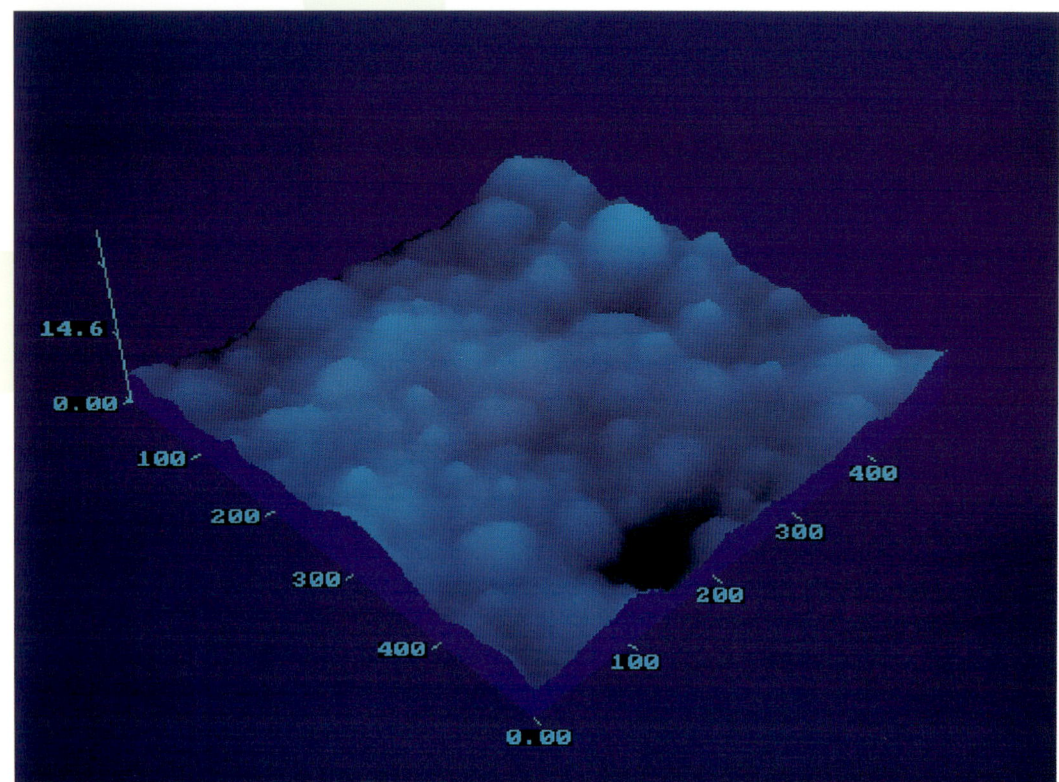

AFM image of crystalline barium titanate
Generally barium titanate is hardly crystallized in normal thin film processings. Either high substrate temperature over 800 K or post-annealing in a high temperature furnace is necessary for crystallizing deposited films. Using ion bombardment onto the growing film surface, we succeeded in depositing barium titanate crystalline film at substrate temperature below 600 K. The AFM image showed the small crystalline particles within 100 nm.

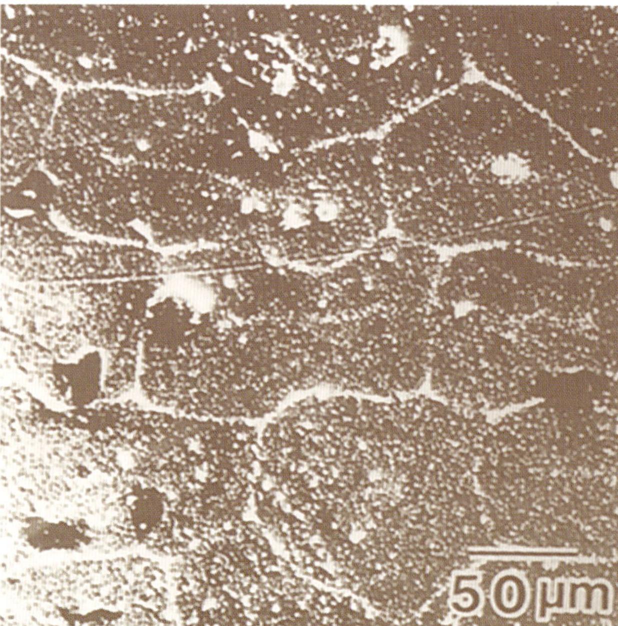

Hydrogen distribution in a high strength steel
Example of SEM-ARG is shown. Tritium was charged in high-strength chromium molybdenum steel, and the specimen was covered by photographic emulsion. After three months exposure, the specimen was developed and the decayed tritium positions were marked by silver particles. Three kinds of hydrogen distributions were observed, namely networks, large particles and small particles inside the networks.

Development of methods for determining the correct position of the atoms (or ions) contained in certain substances plays an important role both for the improvement of the substance and the creation of novel substances.

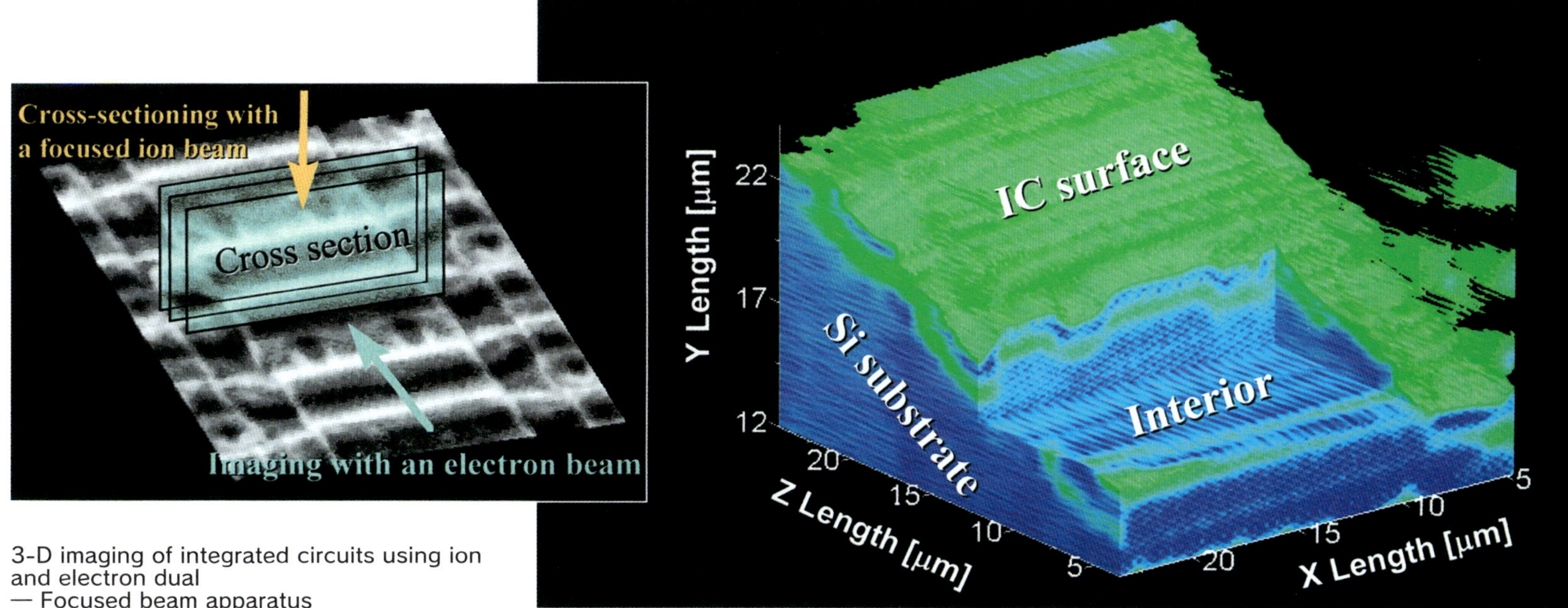

3-D imaging of integrated circuits using ion and electron dual
— Focused beam apparatus

A 3-D analysis method for integrated circuits is required for development and failure analysis. An ion and electron dual-focused beam apparatus has been developed by combining a focused ion beam for micro-cross-sectioning and an electron beam for two-dimensional analysis of the cross-sections. 3-D images of IC patterns and a bonding pad have been observed for the first time.

Cross-sectioning of single microparticle using a focused ion beam

An ion and electron dual-focused beam apparatus for 3-D microanalysis has been developed. This analysis method employs intermittent cross-sectioning of a particle using the focused ion beam and Auger mapping of the cross-sections using the electron beam. 3-D elemental maps are obtained by the repetition of cross-sectioning and Auger mapping under computer control.

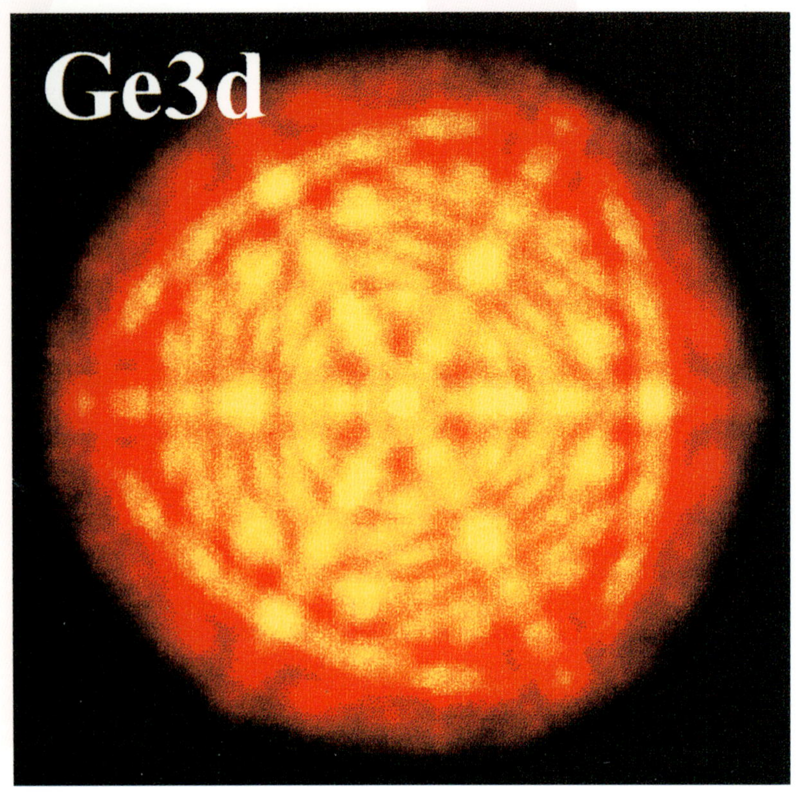

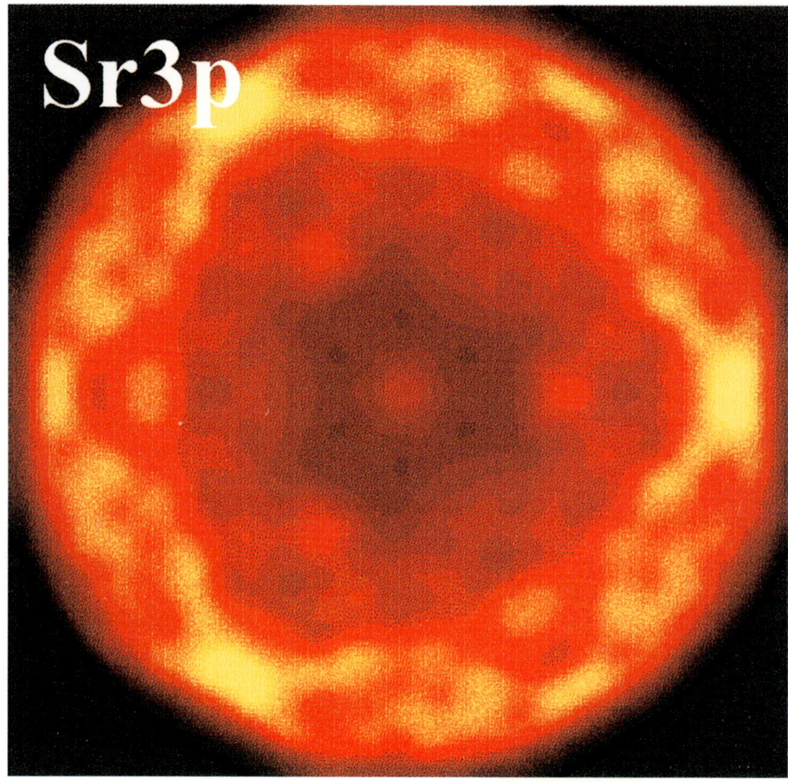

Atomic level characterization of ultrathin films

Atomic level characterization of materials becomes more and more important for the developments of micro-scale devices. X-ray Photoelectron Diffraction (XPED) is a powerful method for analyzing both chemical states and structure of soft materials such as atomically-controlled epitaxial thin films for 3-D electronic devices. Figure shows the XPED patterns from SrF_2 thin films on Ge(111).

Atoms (or ions) consist of the nucleus with a positive charge and the negatively-charged electrons around it. The nature and the positions of the given atoms can be fully characterized by determining the three-dimensional electron-density map precisely.

Atomic surface of high temperature superconductor containing Bi

The superconductor whose electrical resistivity is perfectly 0 has infinite potential for technological applications. The Bi-system superconductor is one of the high-temperature superconductors, having the critical temperature higher than liquid nitrogen ($-192\,^\circ\mathrm{C}$). Bi atoms separated by 0.54 nm are discriminated one by one, when the surface of this material is subjected to Scanning Tunneling Microscopy (STM).

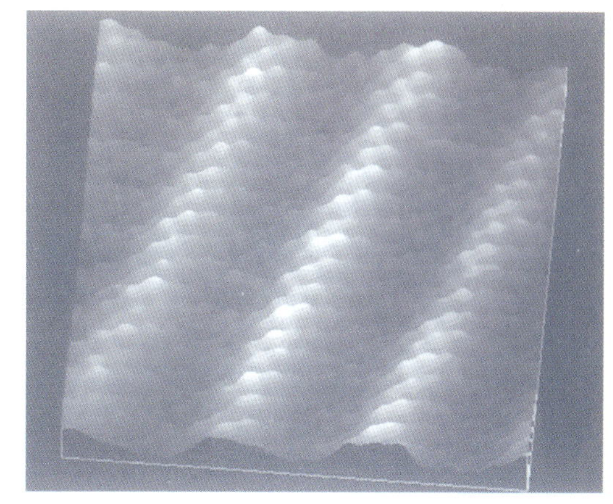

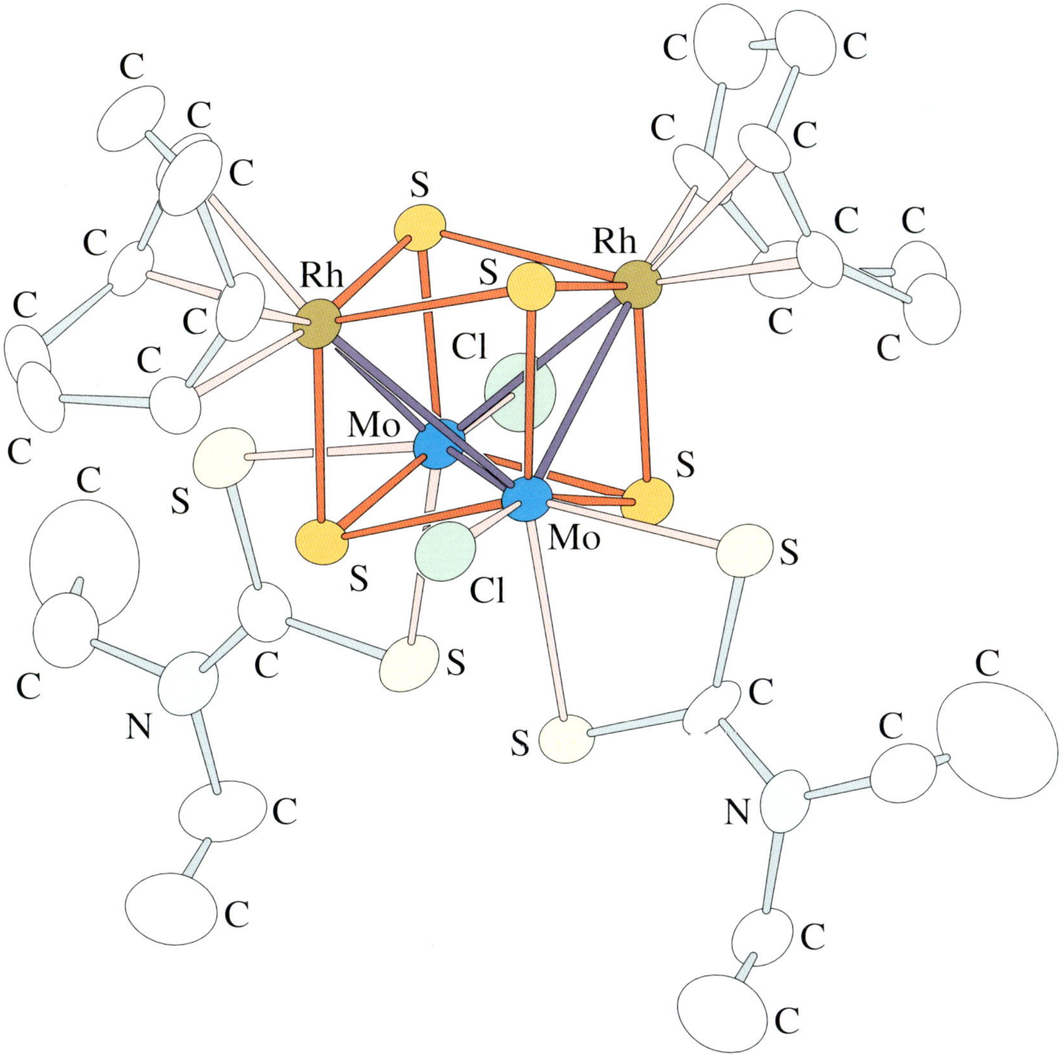

Molecular structure of transition metal–sulfur compound determined by X-ray diffraction study

Analysis of the diffraction map obtained by irradiating a minute single crystal with a monochromated X-ray reveals the detailed structure of the compound involved in the crystal, where the interatomic distance can be expressed in $10^{-13}\,\mathrm{m}$. The figure illustrates the molecular structure of the compound containing a distorted cubic core composed of the transition metals and sulfur atoms, which have been synthesized as the structural model for the active sites of certain metalloenzymes and industrial catalysts.

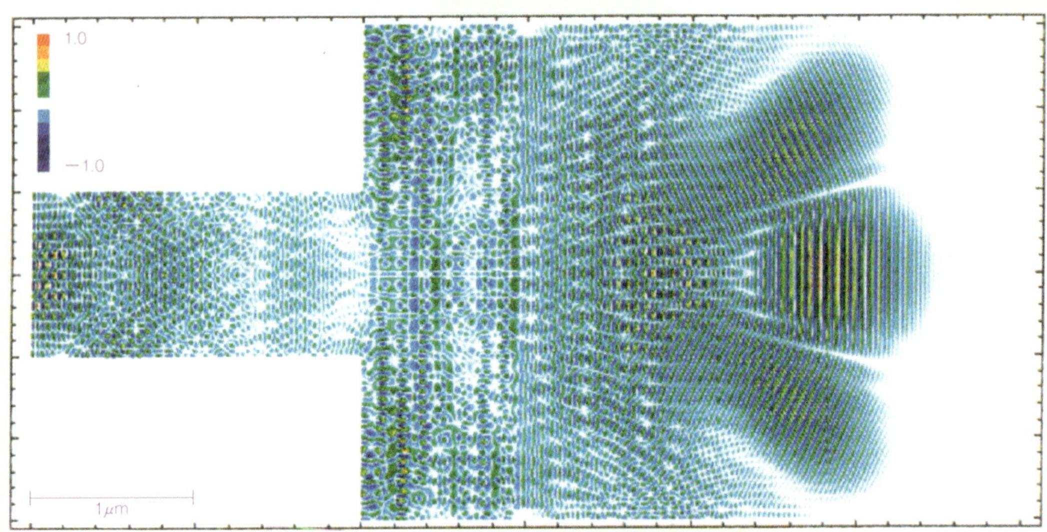

Interference of electron waves in semiconductors

Electrons behave both as particles and waves. Various features of wave natures have been investigated in I.I.S. since 1973, and their device potential explored. The interference of electron waves confined in small semiconductor structures is one example. To clarify this effect, the interference of the electron waves is studied by the computer simulation, as shown in the figure.

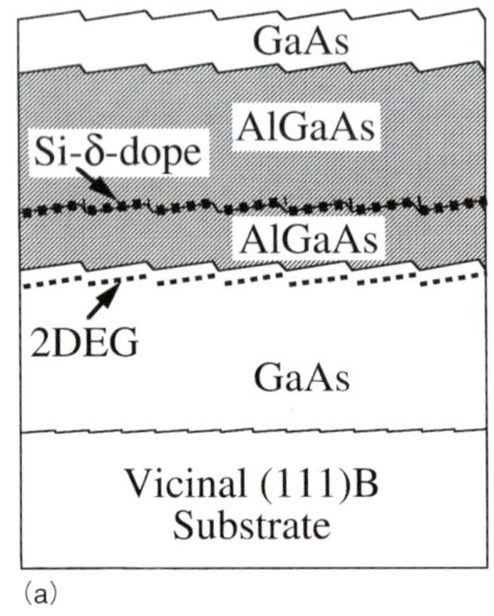

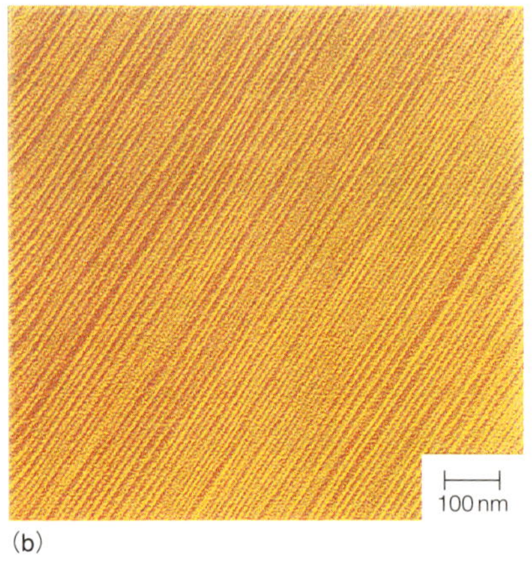

Contol of periodic atomic steps on semiconductors and 10 nm scale quantum wires

Semiconductors (GaAs) grown on a misoriented substrate often exhibit quasi-periodic corrugation originating from atomic steps. Atomic force microscope studies show that steps on tilted (111) GaAs plane are 1.8 nm in height and 15 nm in period. If a conductive layer is formed with such step structures, electrons easily flow only along the steps. Structures in which electrons move only along one direction are called quantum wires. Pioneering research on quantum wires and boxes started in 1975 in IIS, and this opened a new field in solid-state physics and electronics.

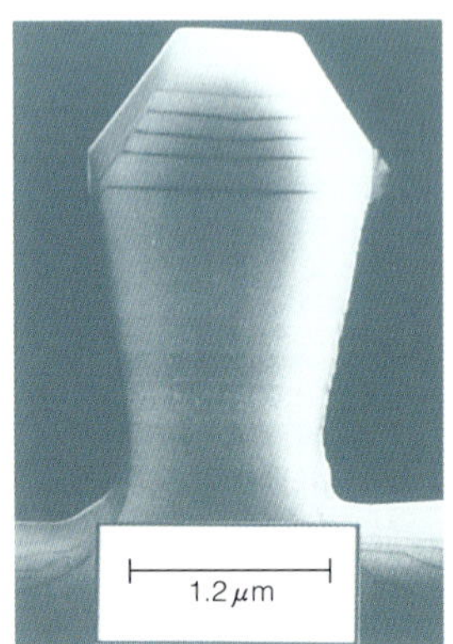

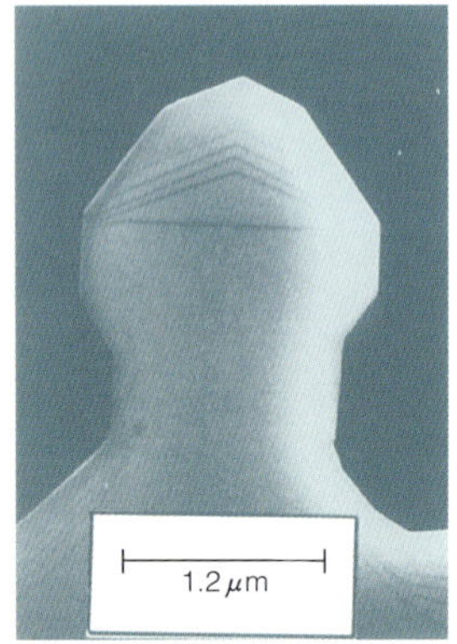

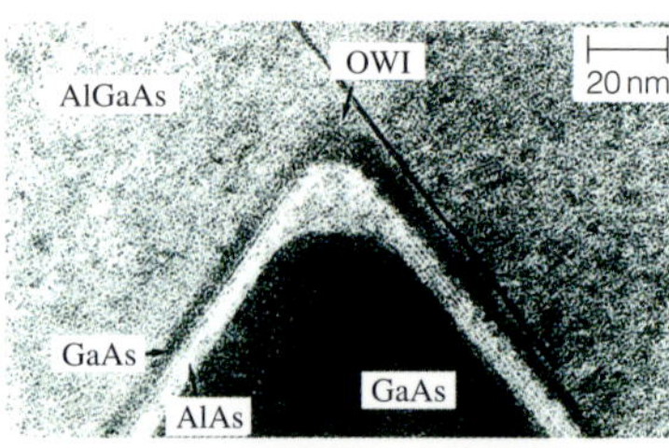

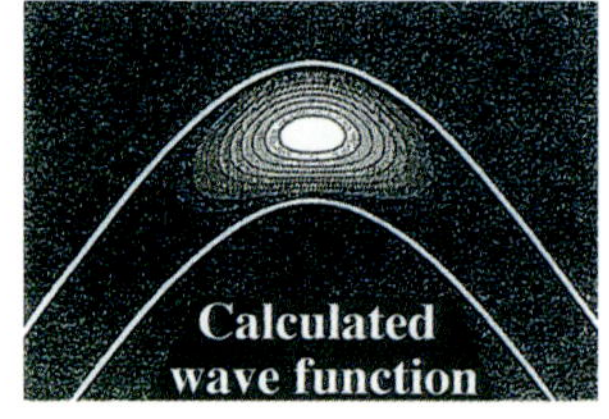

Facet growth of semiconductors and 10 nm scale quantum wires

The epitaxial growth of semiconductor (GaAs or AlAs) on a patterned substrate results in various structures defined by specific crystal planes (facets). The two left figures show such examples of well-defined ridge or roof structures. 10 nm scale quantum wires can be fabricated near the top region of the ridge by depositing a very thin GaAs layer, as electrons are quantum mechanically confined, as shown in the right figures.

GaAs quantum dot in the 2-D photonic crystal using selective growth

We demonstrate the fabrication of quantum dot structures using selective growth by MOCVD. The figures are SEM photographs of the 2-D V-grooves (2-D photonic crystal) and the cross section of GaAs quantum dots at the bottom of the grooves.

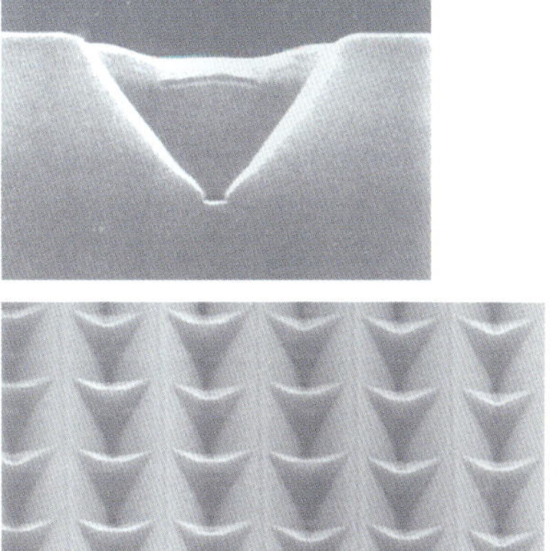
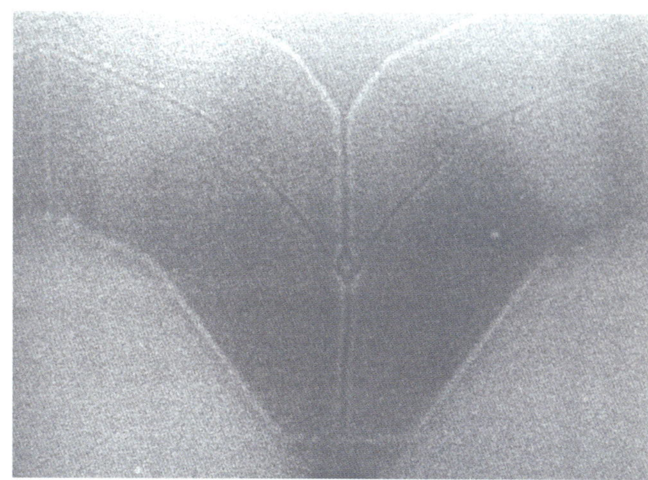

Nano-electronics and nano-optoelectronics

It is important to develop new opto-electronic devices in which interactions between electrons and photons are controlled. For this purpose, fabrication technology for nano-structures plays a key role. The figure shows an SEM picture of a two-dimensional array of GaAs quantum dot structures grown by selective MOCVD.

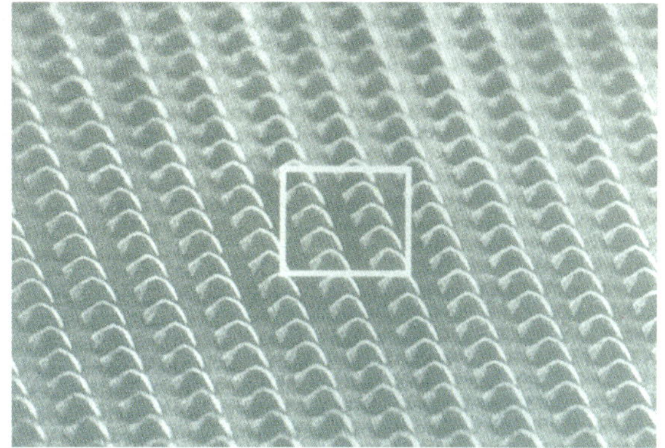
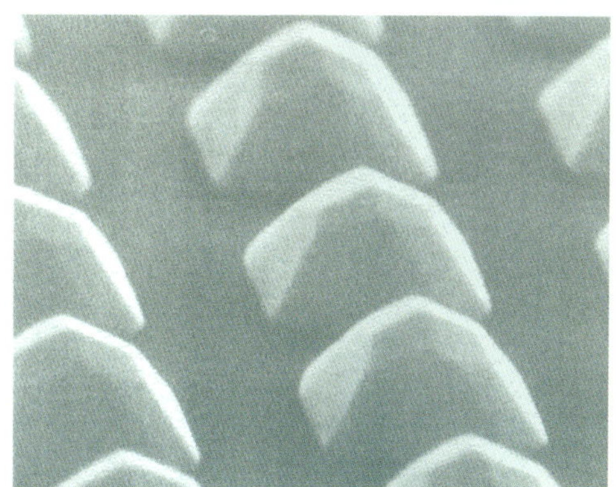

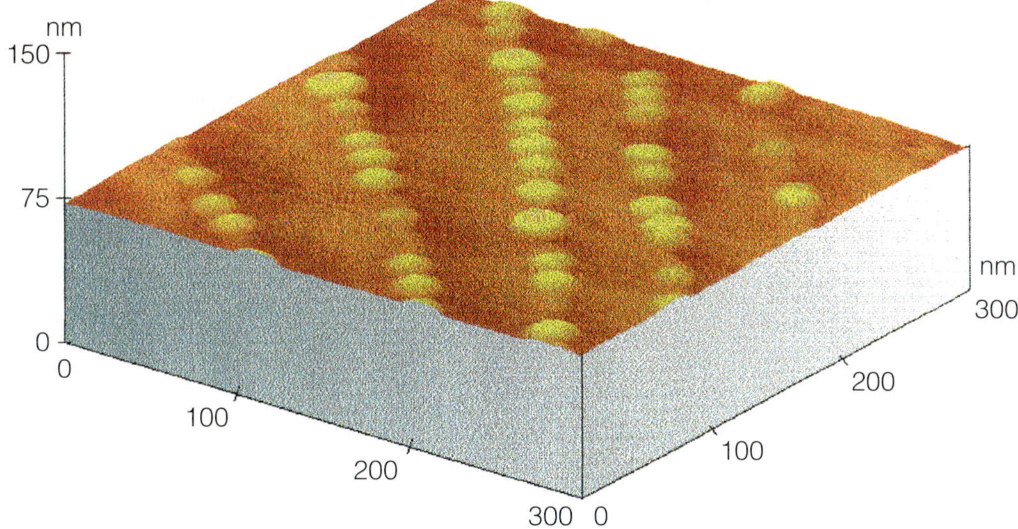

Self-ordering of quantum dots

Fabrication of quantum dots is important for optoelectronic device applications. We fabricated self-assembled InGaAs quantum dots as small as 20 nm on GaAs surface by MOCVD using Stranski-Krastanow growth mode. This method utilized the mismatch of lattice-constants of both deposition and surface material. We successfully controlled the position of InGaAs quantum dots on GaAs. The figure shows the AFM image of naturally ordered InGaAs quantum dots at multi-atomic step edges of surface.

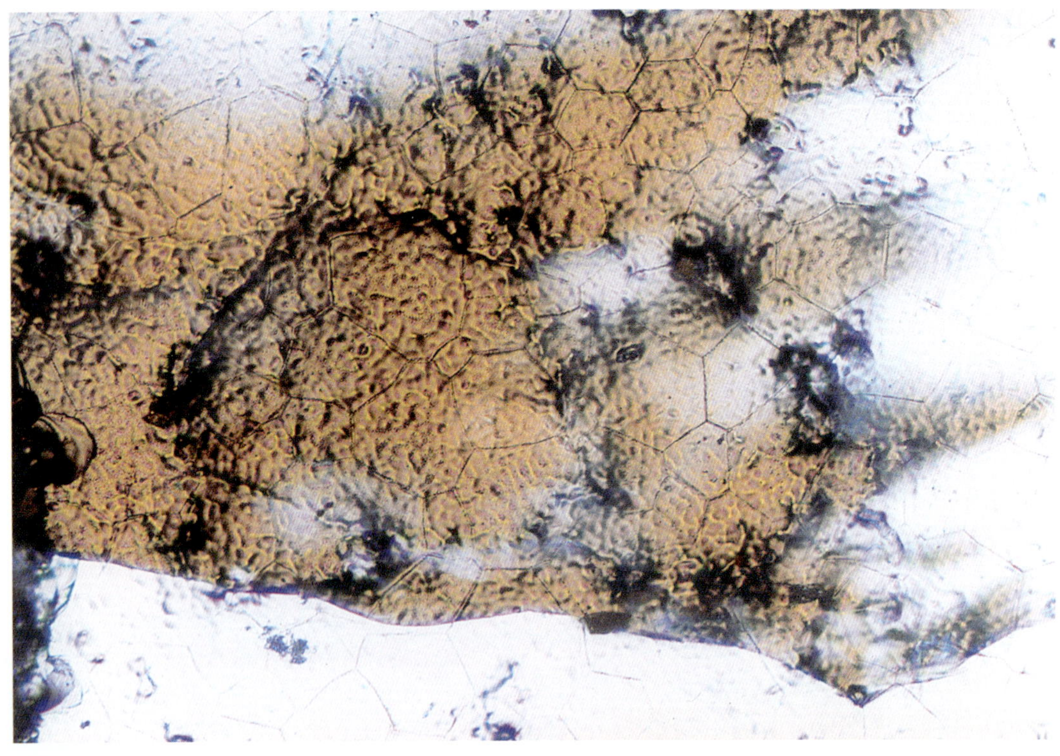

3-D direct observation of fracture behavior in ceramics

Micro-fracture behavior inside ceramic materials is important for the understanding of the fracture mechanism. A new technique has been developed for 3-D direct observation. The photograph shows crack growth behavior from a notch root observed in transparent ZrO_2 (Zirconia). Brown areas in the photograph show cracks inside the material. The photograph clearly demonstrates the difference in fracture behavior between the surface and inside of the material.

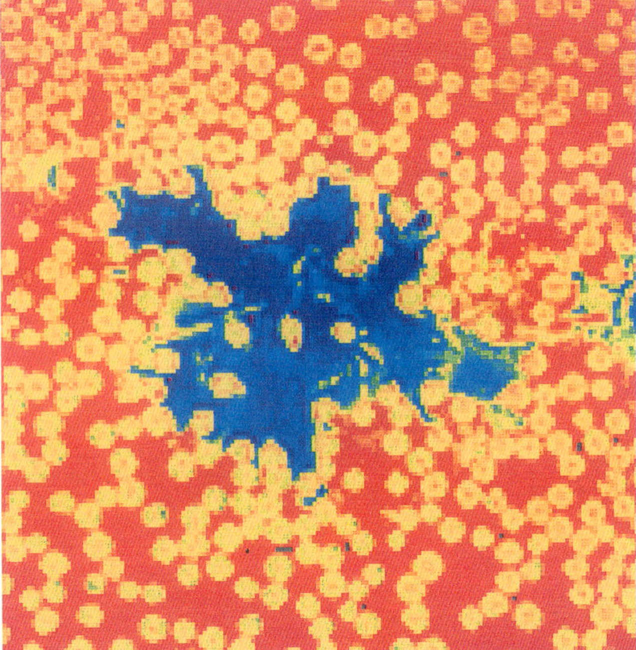

Micro-fracture behavior of a matrix in silicon carbide fiber-reinforced glass matrix composite

Silicon Carbide (SiC) fiber-reinforced glass matrix composite has been expected to be a high temperature lightweight material. The matrix cracking of composite plays an important role in the total performance of the composite. The photograph shows the evolution of the micro-fracture behavior of the matrix by tensile test. The photograph is obtained by the thin-specimen light-transmission method and image analyses. The figure reveals that the cumulative fracture process of the matrix proceeds from a matrix rich area.

Evolution of micro-fracture behavior in silicon carbide fiber-reinforced silicon carbide matrix composite

High fracture resistance of a woven fabric continuous Silicon Carbide (SiC) fiber-reinforced Silicon Carbide (SiC) matrix composite is achieved by the cumulative micro-fracture process of fiber, matrix and interface. The photograph shows a lot of transverse micro cracking, which was introduced during the tensile fracture process. The understanding of micro-fracture behavior is also important in understanding creep and fatigue properties of the composite from room to high temperatures.

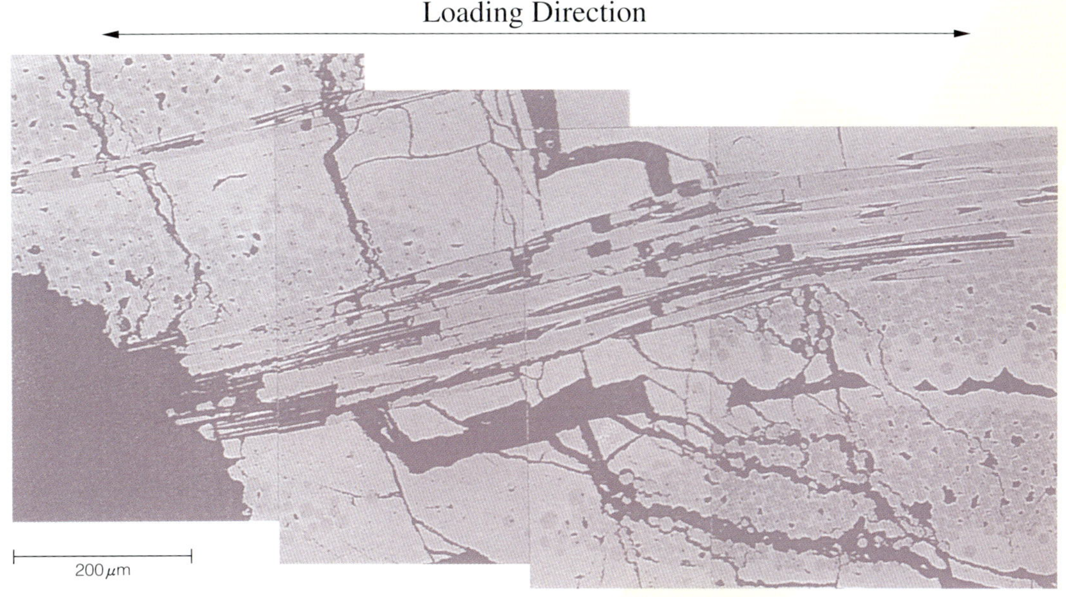

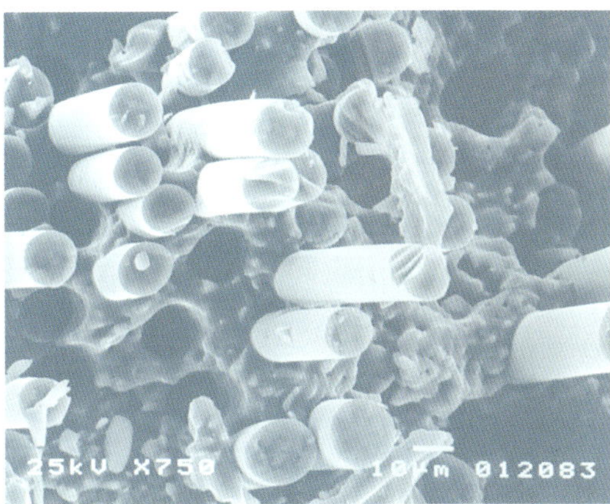

A new approach of interface design in all non-oxide ceramic fiber-reinforced ceramic matrix composite by coating free concept

Control of interface mechanical properties is becoming an important subject of research in the field of continuous fiber-reinforced ceramics. The figure shows the tensile fracture surface of a silicon carbide base SiTiCO fiber-reinforced Silicon Carbide (SiC) matrix composite. Extensive fiber pullout can be observed and this evidence suggests the possibility of a coating-free interface by the surface modification of the fiber.

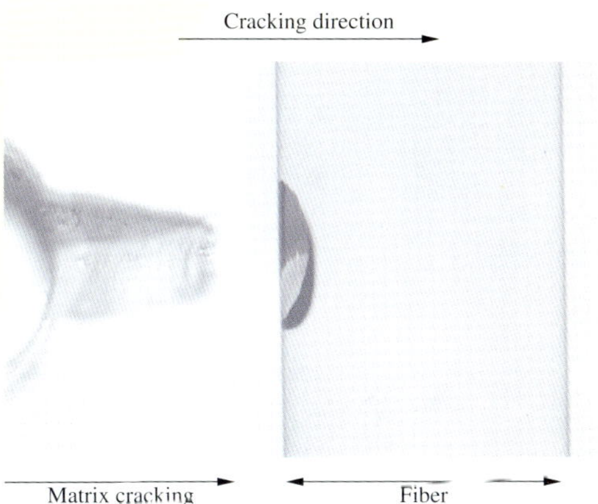

Crack-iterface-fiber interaction process in fiber-reinforced composite-Model experiment

The toughening of fiber-reinforced composites is achieved by the addition of a micro-fracture mechanism. The photograph shows the crack-interface-fiber interaction process. The interface between fiber and matrix ahead of the growing matrix crack is partially debonded. The fundamental result is important in learning the effect of 3-D interaction mechanisms on the properties of fiber-reinforced composites.

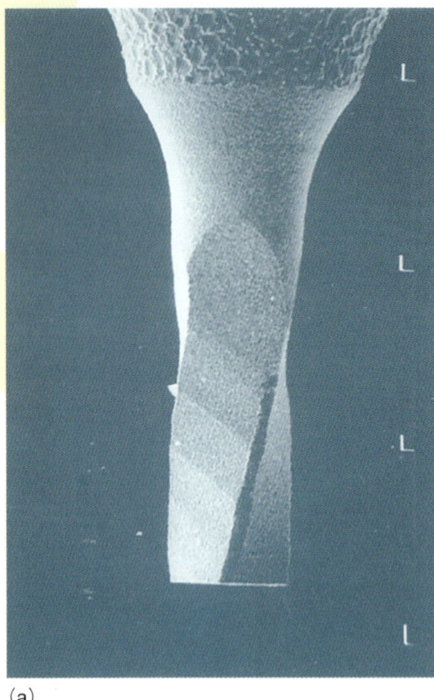

(a)

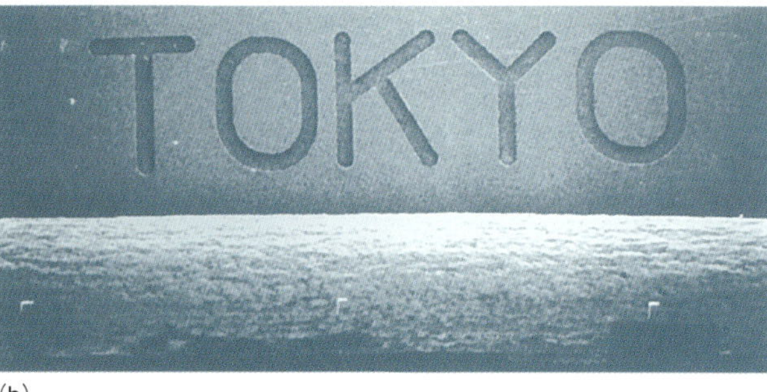

(b)

Milling of microgrooves

Grooves and complex 3-D shapes are often machined by endmilling. It is a difficult problem to apply this to microgrooves with a sufficiently accurate microtool setting. The figures show an example of flat endmill (fig. (a), 50 µm in diameter) and microgrooves (fig. (b), 50 µm of groove width), achieved by on-the-machine tool making using the technique of Wire Electrodischarge Grinding (WEDG).

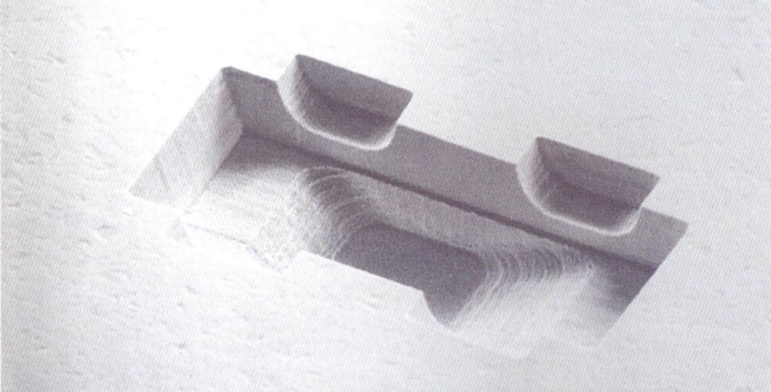

(a)

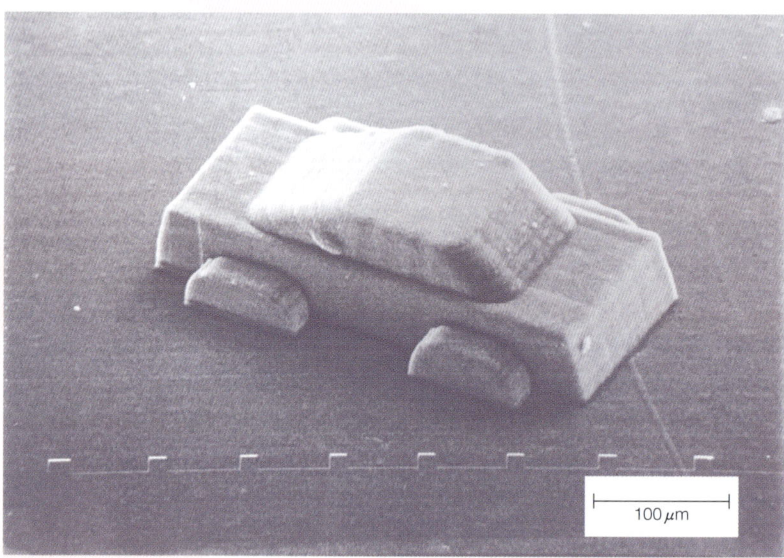

(b)

Micro-EDM for micromolding

Mass production of microparts often requires micromolds. However, the low strength and/or high wear rate of tools have been a barrier to fabricating micromolds by cutting or EDM. In order to solve these problems, an EDM system was developed in which a simple shape electrode is scanned along a specially designed path. This system was proved to be free from the electrode wear problem. Figures show a micromold (fig. (a)) produced by this system, and a molded plastic model (fig. (b)).

When we look around carefully, we can see that there are minute three-dimensional shapes, such as the organization of our own skin. In order to create such microstructures, it is necessary to devise them using non-conventional methods.

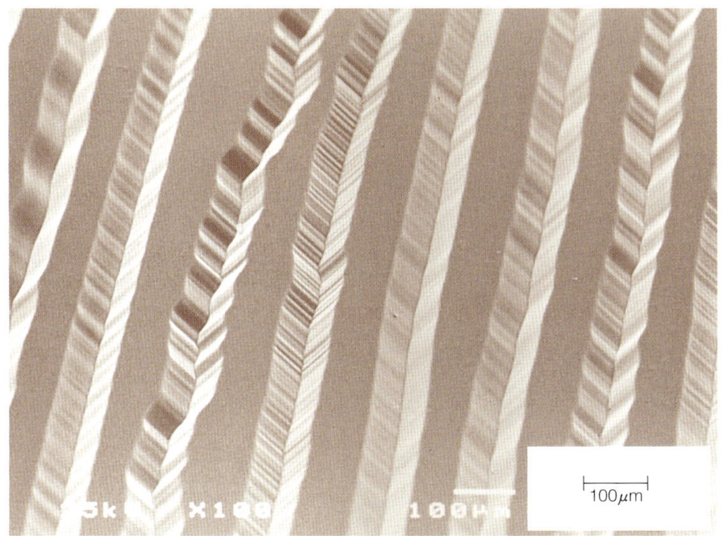

(a)

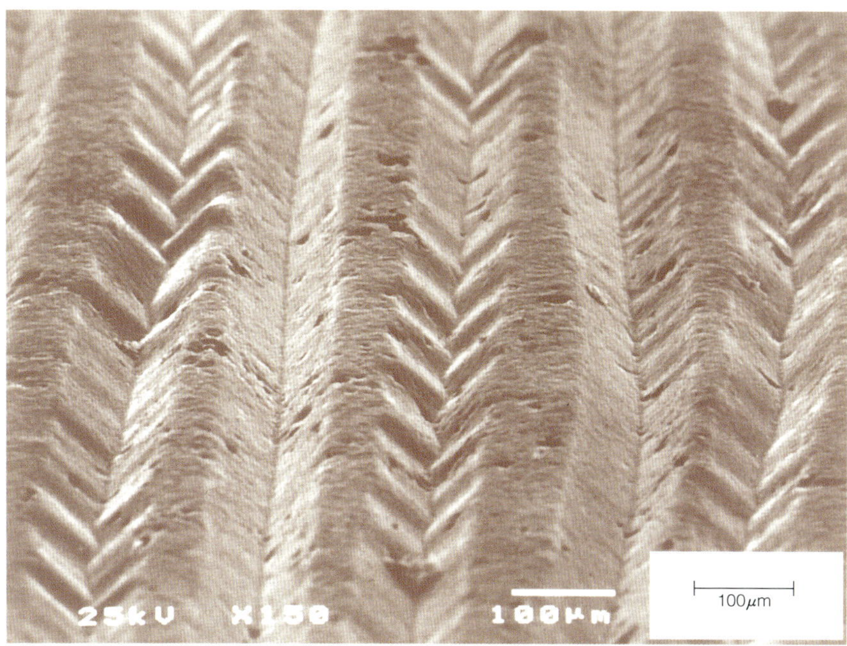

(b)

Aluminum alloy record disc produced by ultra-precision casting

A cast-metal record disc was produced as an experiment to find ultimate precision in metal casting. A casting sand (fine ceramic powder) mold surface was transferred from the real record disc (fig. (a)), and a molten aluminum alloy is cast into the mold while air was being sucked through it (fig. (b)). The music can be enjoyed despite the presence of slight noise.

Lapping stone including microcapsules

We developed a lapping stone including microcapsules which contained perfluoropolyether oil having a tribochemical reaction on workpiece. From the lapping results, it was confirmed that the tribochemical reaction between the oil and the workpiece surface was generated and it resulted in a significant improvement of the finishing efficiency and the surface quality of aluminum workpieces, as well as silicon wafers.

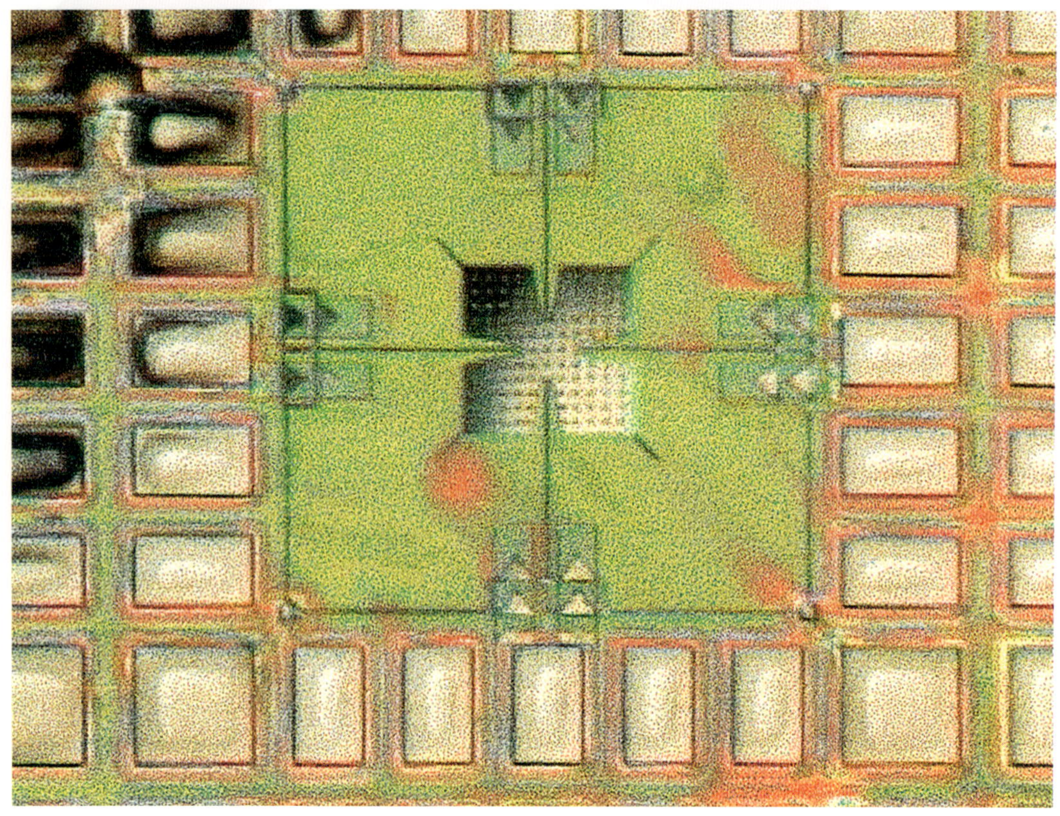

Micro X-Y stage driven by scratch drive actuators

The device shown in the figure is the micro-optical stage to control the beam axis or the focusing depth. Microactuators (for generating force, the triangle parts in the figure) were developed by the silicon micromachining technique. The actuators push or pull the stage tethered with the suspensions. The size of the stage is 0.3 mm by 0.3 mm, and the displacement was 0.1 mm.

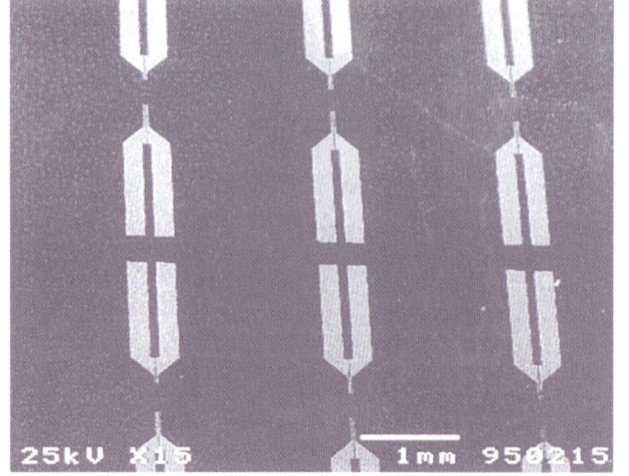

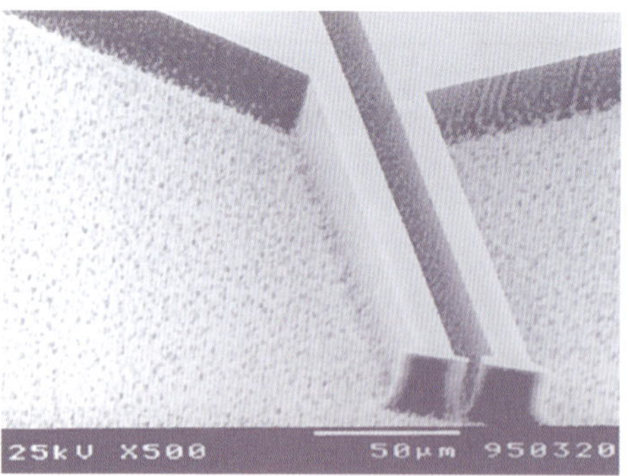

Micro twin probes for the vibroscanning method, with a close-up on the picture

It was technically possible to make such tiny holes that even a hair could not pass through. However, no measurement technique has been available so far to investigate the size or smoothness of the holes. We have developed probes which look like the sensing hair of an insect, by using the silicon micromachining technique. Inserting the dithering probe into the hole, we could detect the profile of the hole at the moment of the probe touching the wall surface. The probe could be scanned around or along the hole to see the profile.

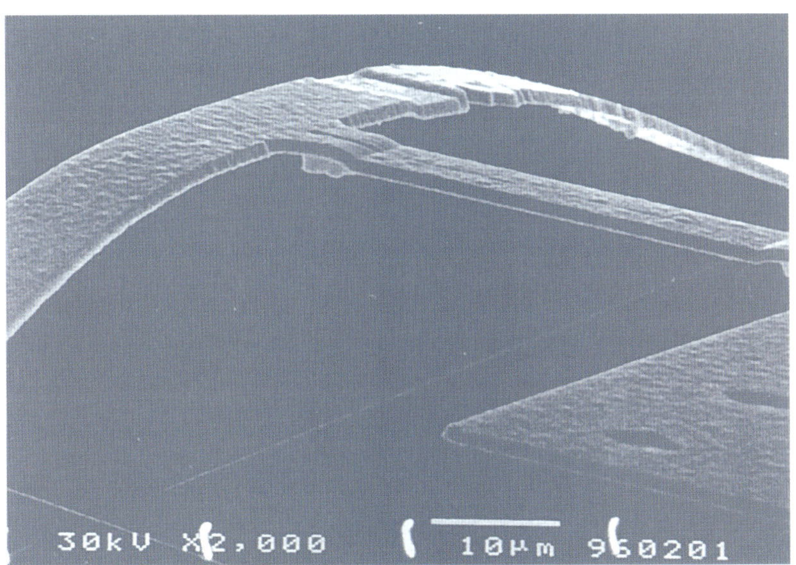

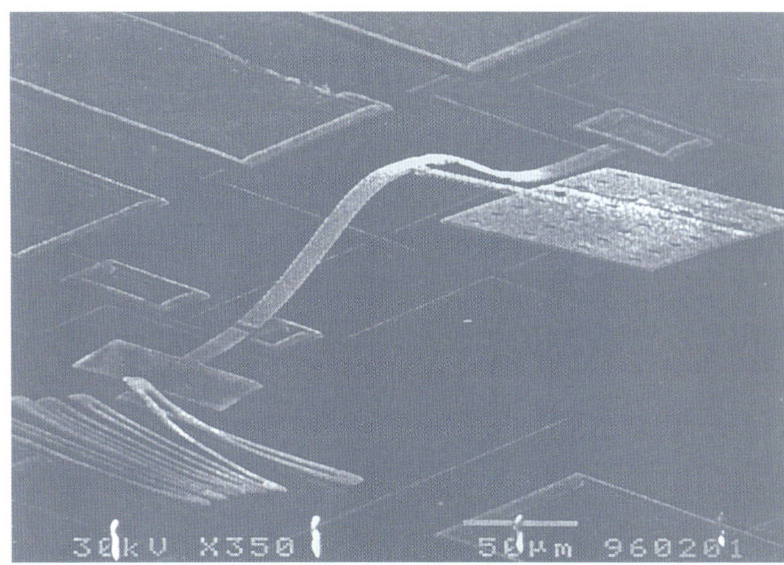

Poly-Si 3-D micro structures

A new process, called "Reshaping Technology", was developed to fabricate three-dimensional micro structures. First, a flat polysilicon structure was made by surface micromachining. A micro actuator raised it in the vertical direction to the substrate. The 3-D shape was retained by flowing current, and producing Joule heat on the structure and plastically deforming it.

Micro-machined quartz optical chopper

A resonating chopper for optical sensors was fabricated by photolithography , and anisotropic etching of single crystal quartz. Au/Cr film covers a resonator (4 mm × 2 mm × 0.1 mm) with six windows. The resonator is suspended by four plate springs and driven by the piezoelectric effect of quartz. An expanded view of the spring shows the thin driving electrodes on it.

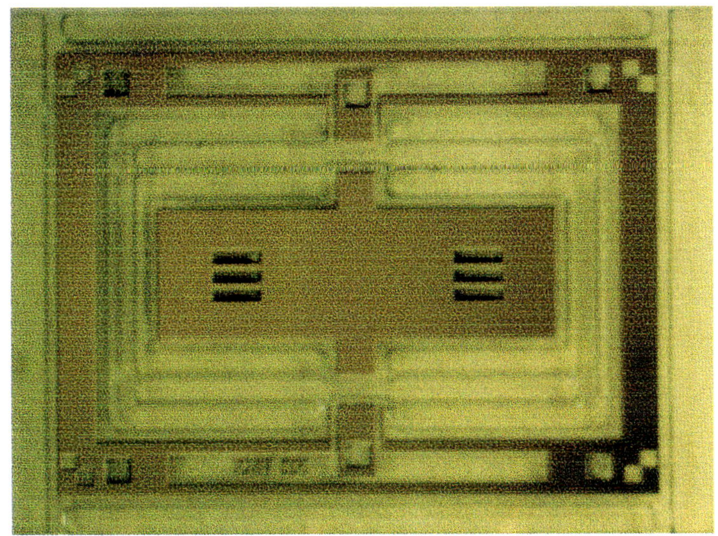

(a)

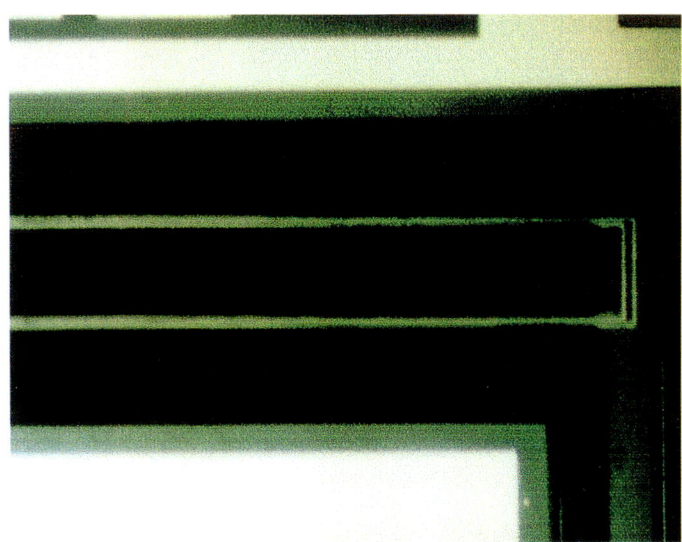

(b)

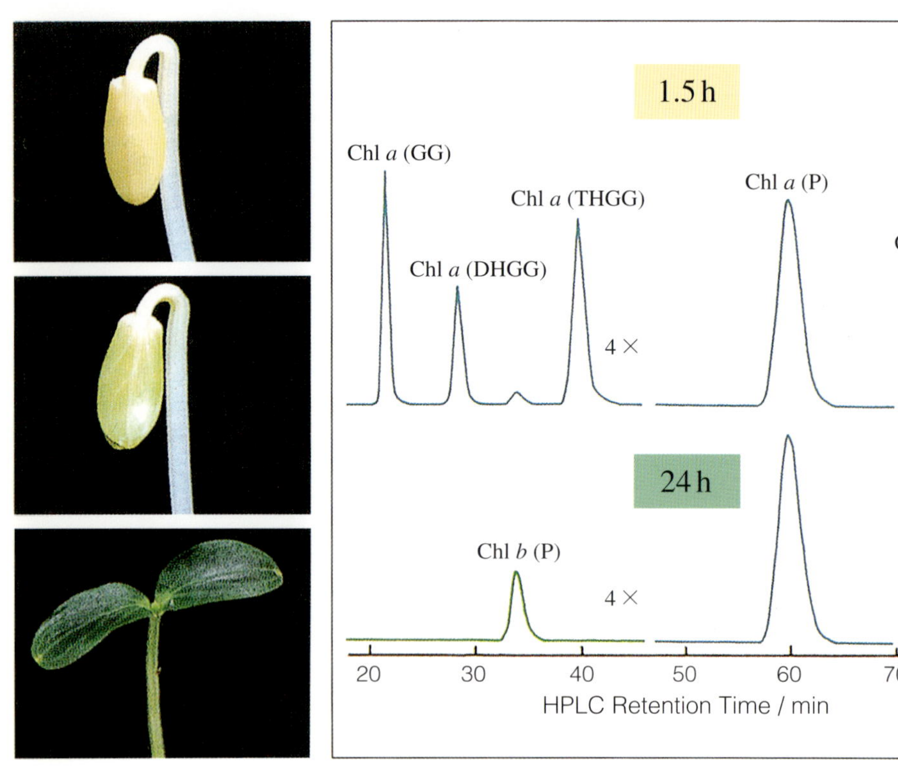

Temporal evolution of photosynthetic molecular assembly during greening of etiolated leaves

To elucidate the molecular assembly of photosynthetic organs, the in-vivo pigment composition during greening of cucumbers is studied here, by quantifying a minor but key pigment (chlorophyll a' (Chl a')), two molecules of which have been detected by ourselves in the very near vicinity of the so-called reaction center I of higher plants, algae, and cyanobacteria.

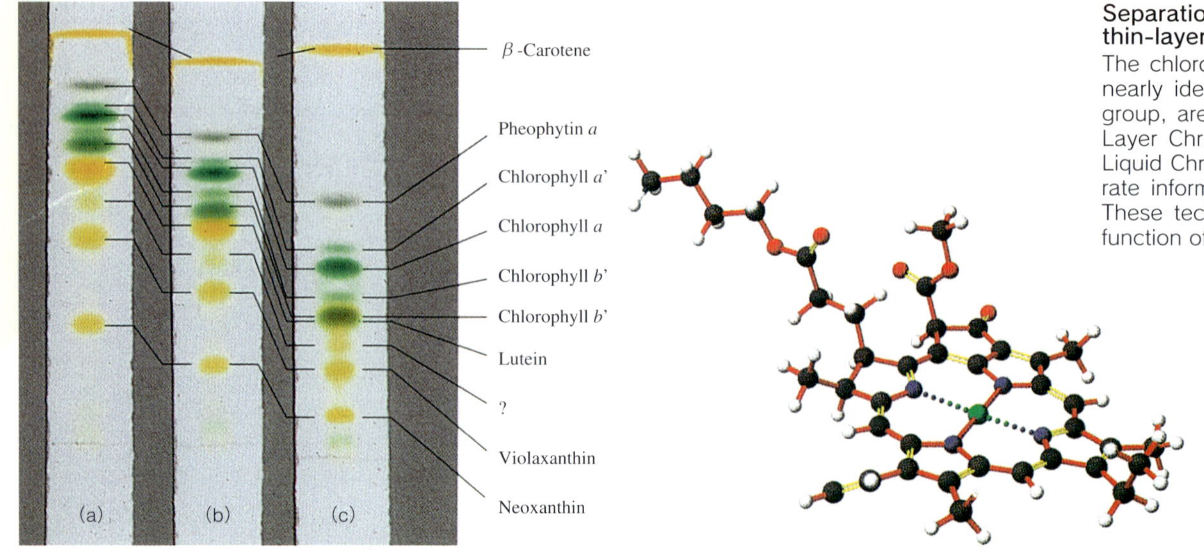

Separation of photosynthetic pigments by thin-layer chromatography

The chlorophylls and carotenoids, which possess nearly identical molecular structures within each group, are visually separated here by silica Thin-Layer Chromatography (TLC). High-Performance Liquid Chromatography (HPLC) yields more accurate information on the amount of the pigments. These techniques are used to clarify the in-vivo function of chlorophyll a' (inset).

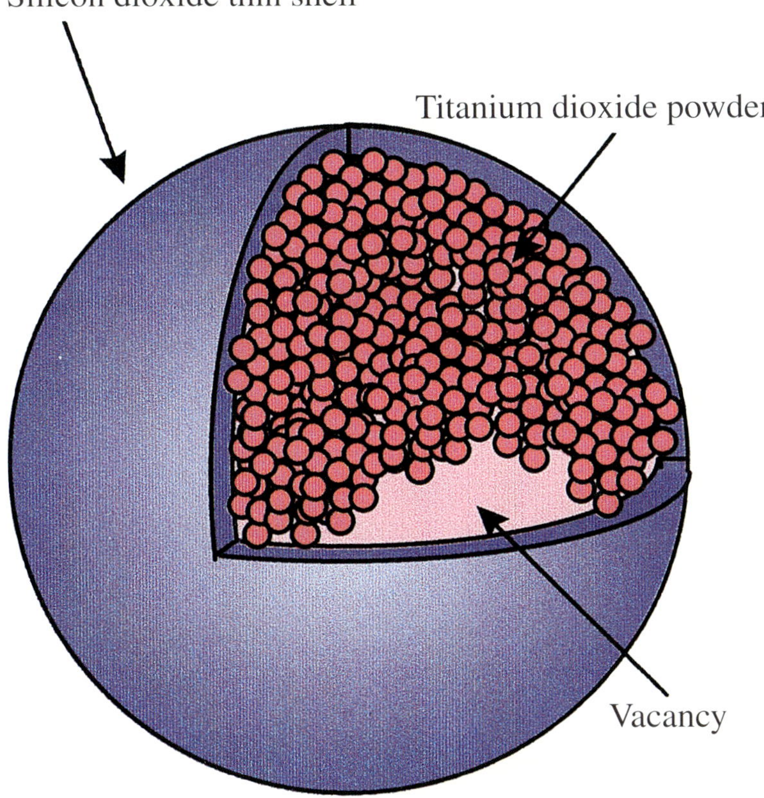

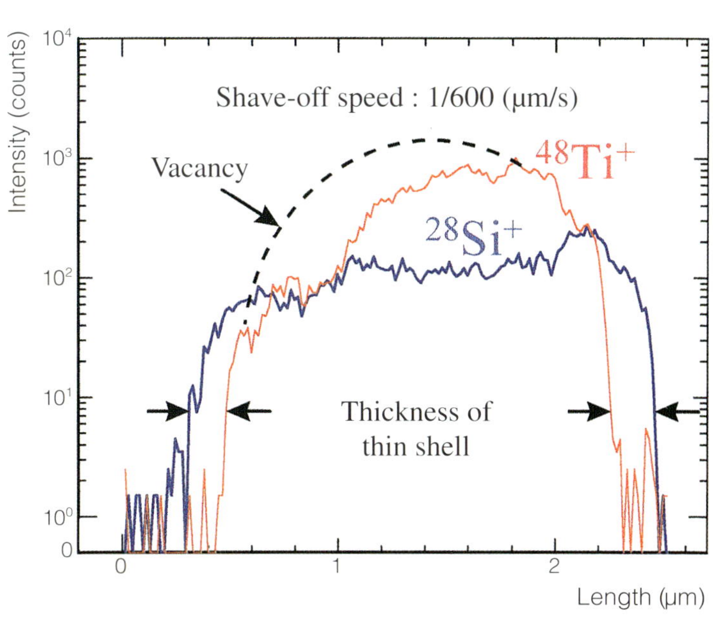

Individual particle analysis of an iorganic microcapsule using a submicron SIMS apparatus

The sample is an inorganic microcapsule, which consists of powder of titanium dioxide inside a thin shell of silicon dioxide. The diameter of this particle is from 2 to 3 μm. A single particle is analyzed by shave-off analysis or 3-D analysis. By these analyses, the thickness of the thin shell (0.04 ~ 0.27 μm), the volume of the internal vacancy (0 ~ 80 vol. %) and the elemental distribution can be measured accurately.

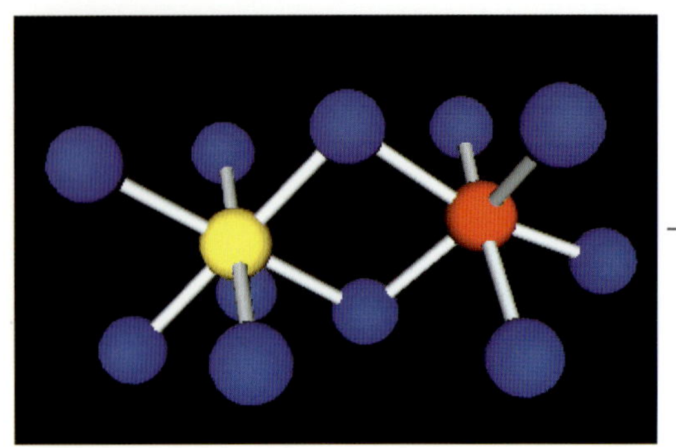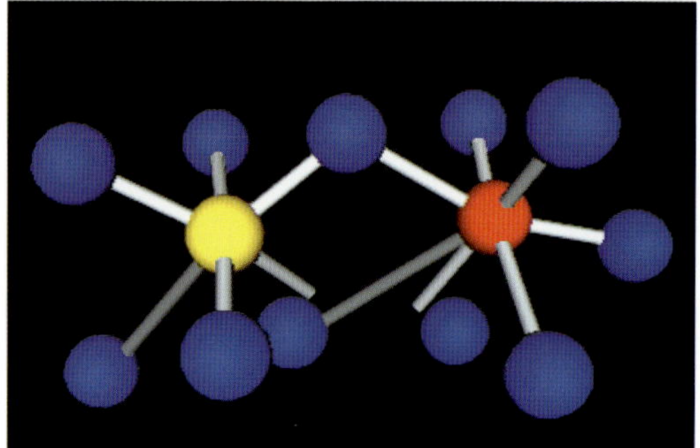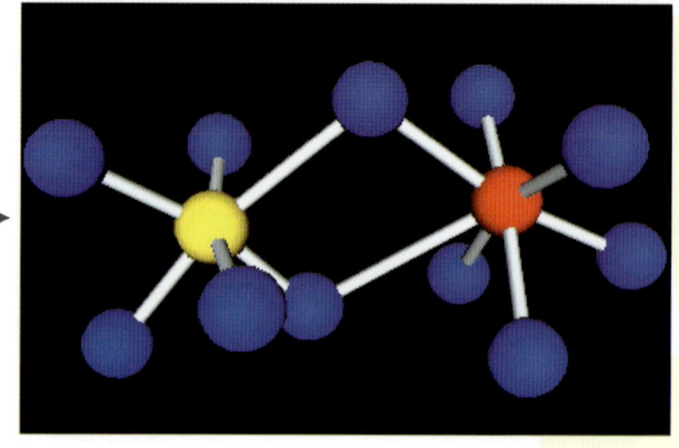

Tin doping mechanism in indium oxide by MD simulation

Tin doped indium oxide (ITO) has been used in a variety of opto-electronic devices. It is necessary to understand the Sn doping mechanism in In_2O_3 to produce higher quality films. In order to investigate the mechanism, the atomic configuration around the doped Sn atoms has been examined by MD (Molecular Dynamics) simulation.

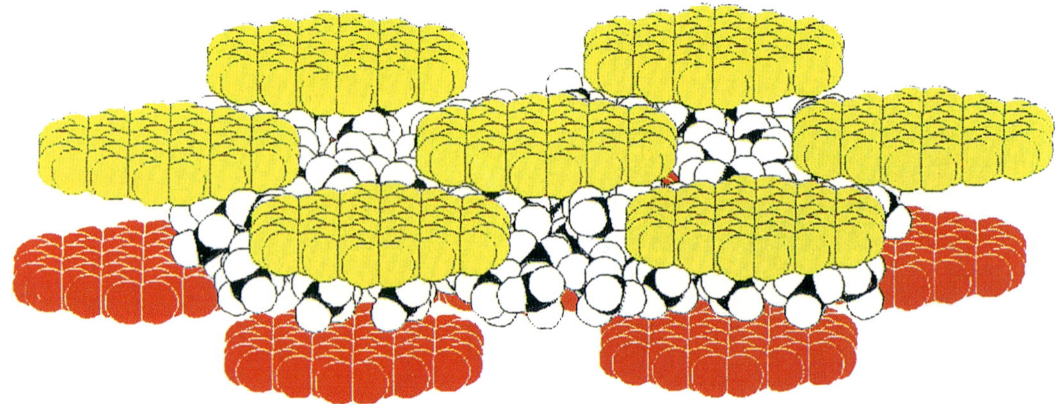

Molecular simulation of methane adsorption onto activated carbon

The proper choice of activated carbon is usually responsible for the performance of the adsorption processes utilizing activated carbon. However, activated carbons are still produced on the basis of empirical knowledge only. In order to establish a methodology for systematically designing customized and the most effective activated carbons for specific applications, molecular simulation models have been developed.

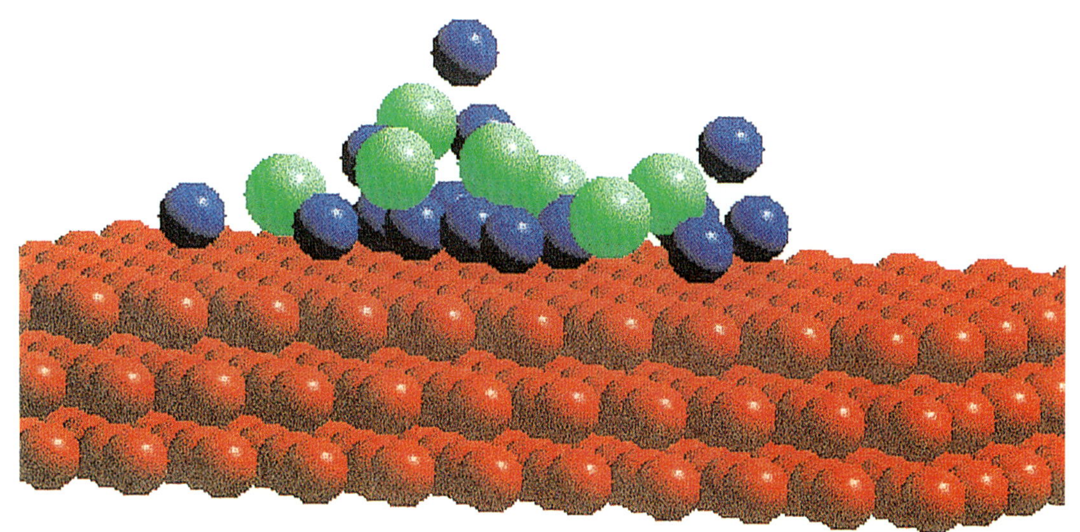

Mechanism of surfactant epitaxy by molecular dynamics

A small amount of pre-adsorbed foreign atoms on the substrate is known to change the growth mode of a film from 3-D island growth to 2-D layer by layer growth. This is called surfactant epitaxy and is expected to be a powerful method of controlling film growth. The figure shows the film growth process by molecular dynamics simulation. This is the growth of Ni (blue) on a Ni surface (red) with pre-adsorbed Pb atoms (green). The growth proceeds by the Ni atoms exchanging their positions with Pb atoms.

The calculation of impurity-induced embrittlement in Al grain boundaries

It has been demonstrated by experiment that a very small amount of impurities in Al tend to segregate at grain boundaries and induce embrittlement. In order to clarify the mechanism of embrittlement, first principles molecular dynamics are used to calculate the electronic and atomic structure. The figure shows the charge density distribution near Al grain boundaries, which indicates the low charge density near grain boundaries (the darker the green, the higher the charge density).

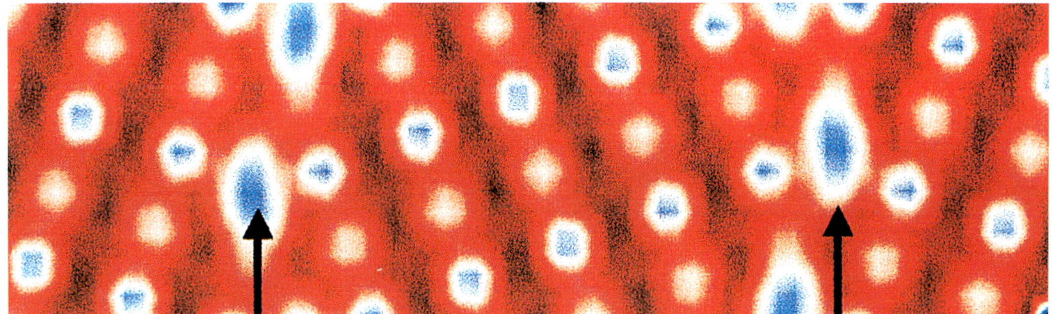

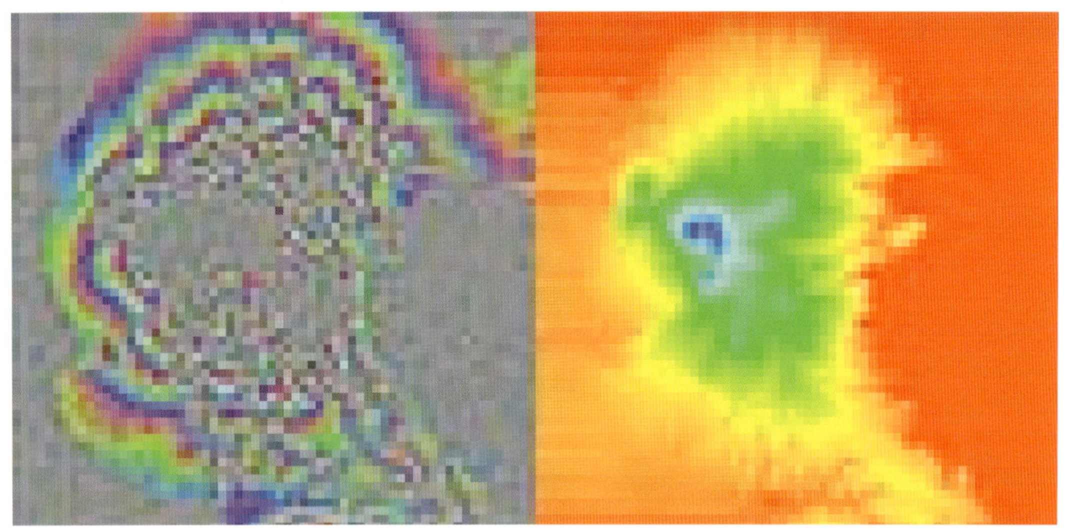

Automated topographical measurements using satellite SAR interferometry

Elevation, which is fundamental to the understanding of the land surface, can be derived using satellite-based remote sensing images. The figure shows an interferogram acquired by satellite remote sensing SAR (Synthetic Aperture Radar) images. The rings of the interferogram represent the ground elevation, and the digital elevation data can be calculated from these.

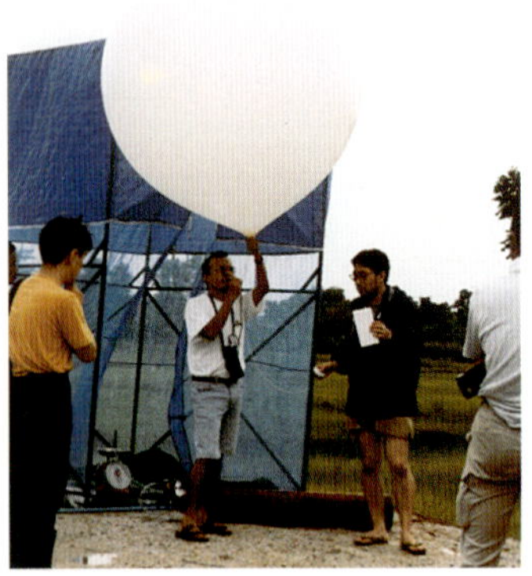

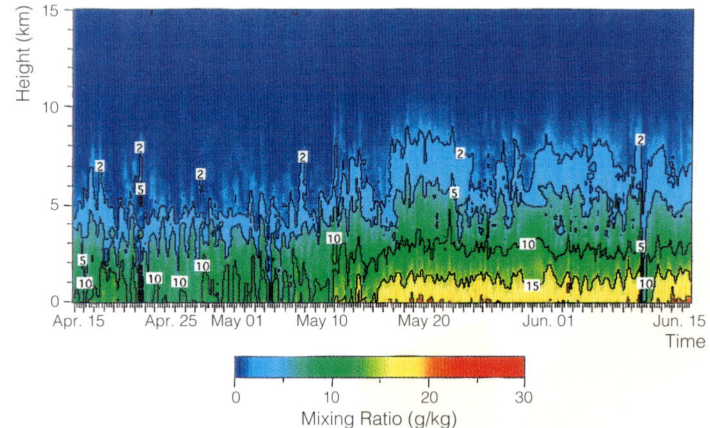

GEWEX Asian monsoon experiment (GAME) in tropics

Tropical areas of south-east Asia influenced by the Monsoon appear to have a common rainy season, but climate and water resources shows pronounced differences between areas due to the effects of topography, latitudinal location and so on. International cooperative experiments, GAME in the tropics, are conducted to investigate the water and energy cycles there. The figure provides the atmospheric profile change at higher temporal resolution than ever.

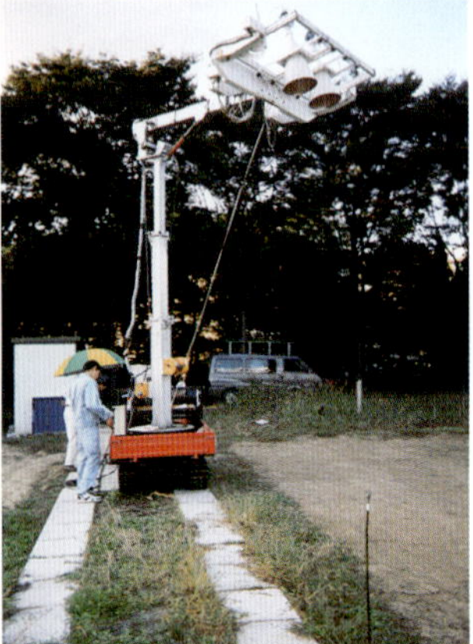

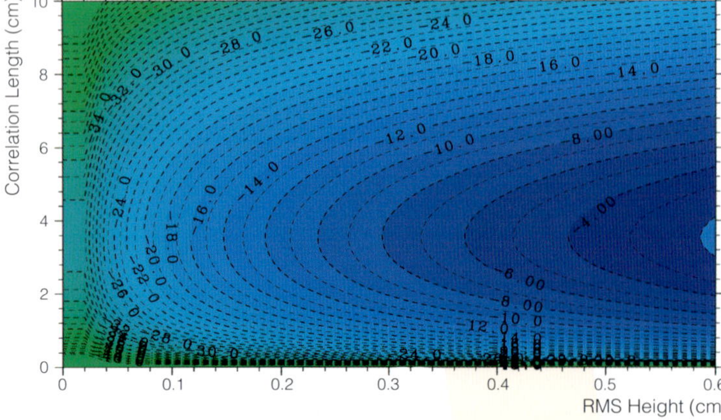

Surface soil moisture measurement using active microwave remote sensing

The surface soil moisture is an important factor controlling the interaction between the Earth's surface and the atmosphere. Space platform-based active microwave remote sensing is expected to measure the soil moisture distribution over a large area. Ground-based experiments including satellite verification are conducted for its practical applications.

Development of early earthquake damage estimation systems for urban lifelines

In order to prevent secondary disasters after an earthquake in the Tokyo Metropolitan area, an emergency shut-off system (SIGNAL) was developed for a large-scale city gas network. The system performs an estimate of the hypocenter and magnitude of the earthquake, and an estimate of damage using the records from a very dense seismic monitoring network. Further research aimed at upgrading the system is still being carried out.

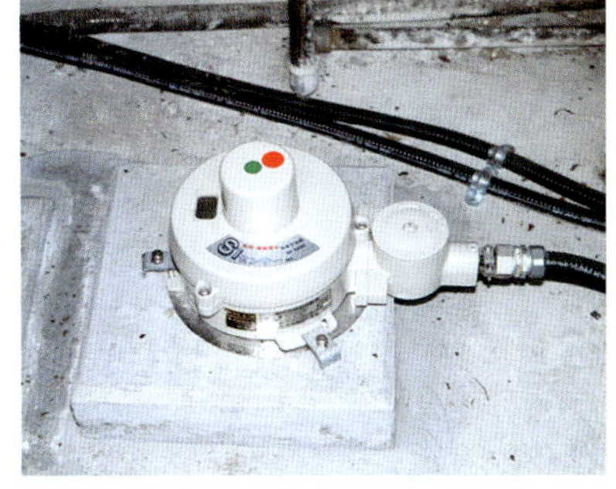

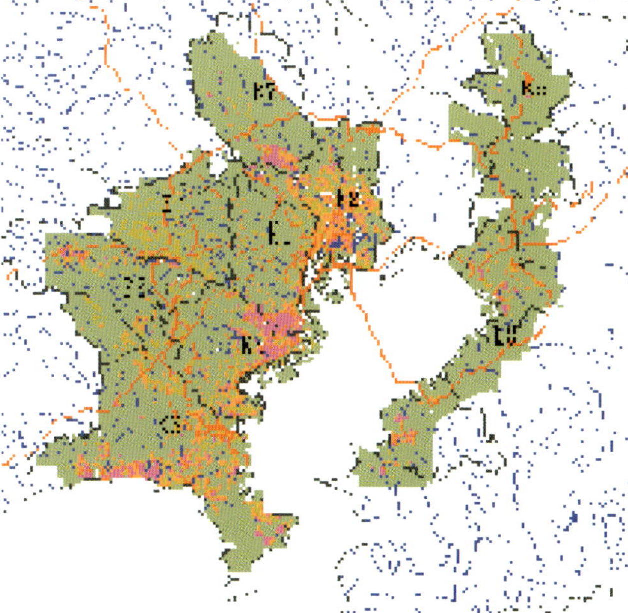

Estimation of the effects of power outage in urban areas in order to determine optimum counter-measures

Lifeline systems such as electric power, water and gas supply systems and telecommunication systems, etc. are the major issues in urban disaster mitigation measures. Our modern societies rely heavily on electric power and suffer functional damage due to power outage when natural disasters such as earthquakes and typhoons strike. In order to develop a new methodology for estimating the effects of power outage on city functions taking account of the characteristics of the area, the occurrence time and duration of the outage, a database is being developed which consists of regional characteristics and the electric power demand in Tokyo using geographic information systems. Using this database, a new methodology for estimating the effects of power outage is proposed, which can be used for optimum disaster mitigation measures before and after an accident. The figure shows the effects when a power stops at 6:00 a.m. (top) and 6:00 p.m. (bottom). It is clear that even the duration of outage is same, its effects become very different due to the difference of regional characteristics.

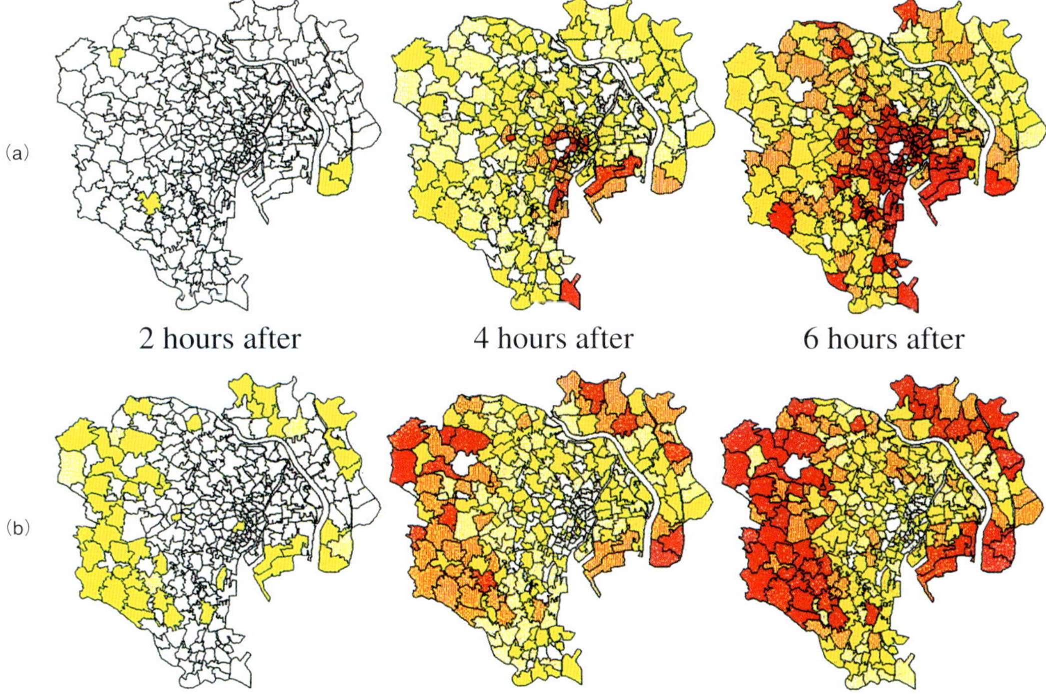

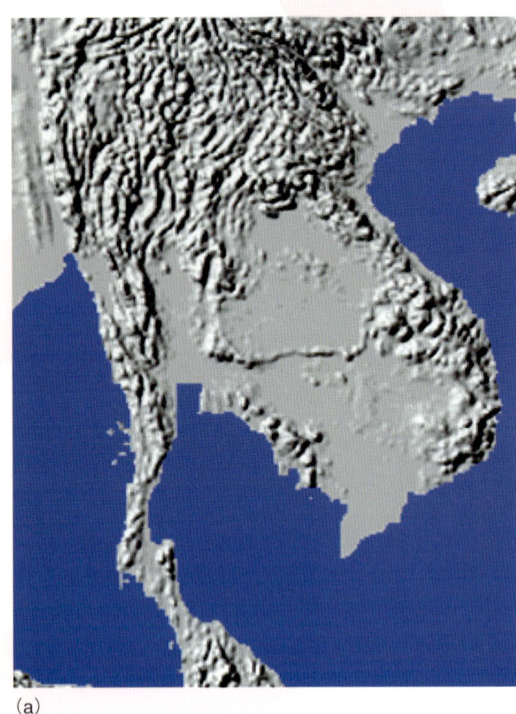

(a)

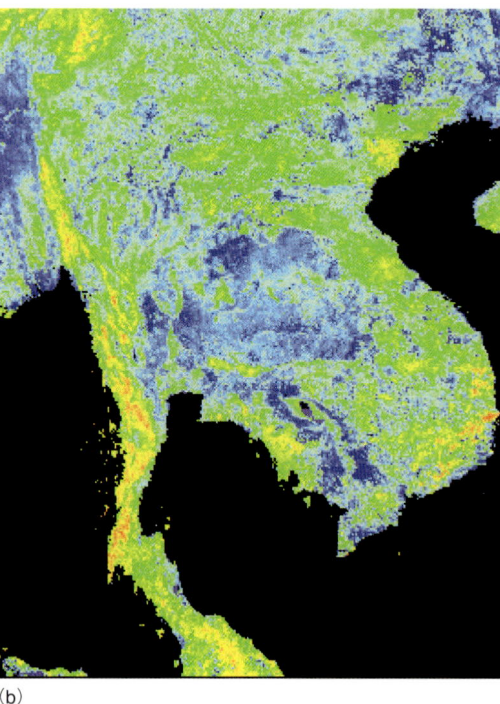

(b)

Remote sensing satellites are sending us huge amounts of data

It is important to develop an effective data management system for Remote Sensing and GIS users. The database is equipped with a parallel processing system to undertake automated geometric correction and classification. Daily received NOAA satellite data (fig. (a)) which accounts for a few gigabytes and global GIS data such as elevation data (fig. (b)) can be stored in our digital geographic data library.

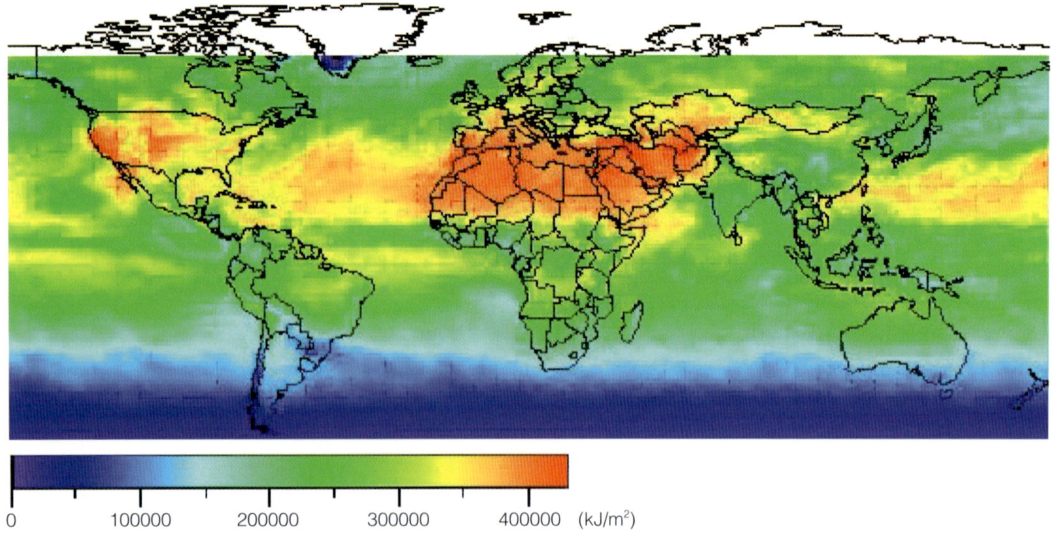

Satellite remote sensing data provides us with various information

The figure shows the annual amount of solar energy, which can be absorbed by inland vegetation, the so-called PAR (Photosynthesis Active Radiation). This figure illustrates how much solar energy is possible to be converted to the NPP (Net Primary Production).

TRIP
— Information on the global river channel network

Total Runoff Integrating Pathways (TRIP), a global river channel network, was developed in 1 degree by 1 degree grid boxes (approximately 100km square) for whole continents. Its accuracy and the reality are well examined, and used for linking meteorological and climatological information to hydrological and water resource-related issues.

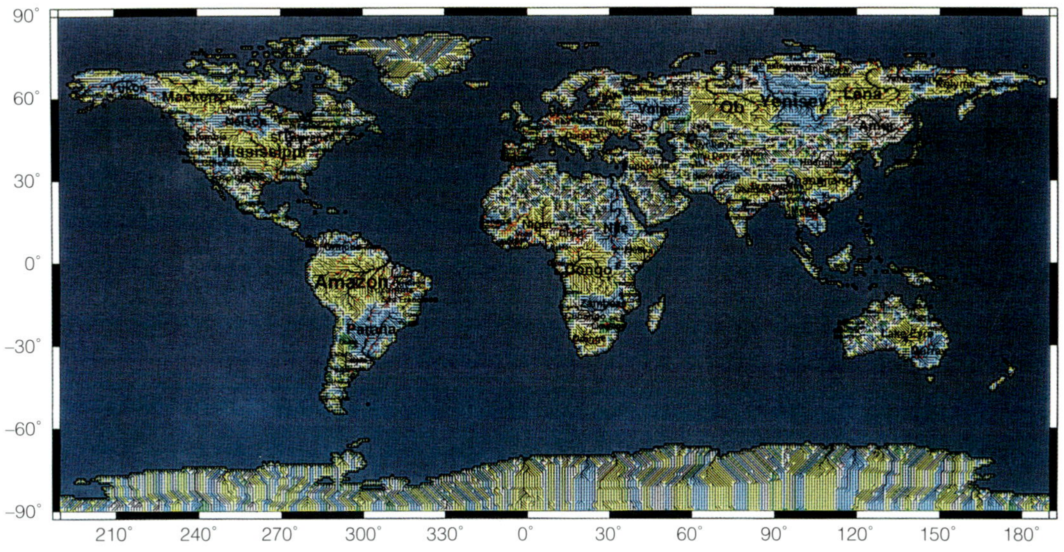

Global distribution of vertically integrated annual water vapor flux convergence

The global distribution of water vapor convergence/divergence field was estimated based on a four-dimensional data assimilation dataset made by the European Centre for Medium-Range Weather Forecasts. According to the atmospheric water balance, the long-term mean of the convergence corresponds to precipitation minus evapotranspiration, and such information is useful in the assessment of global water cycles.

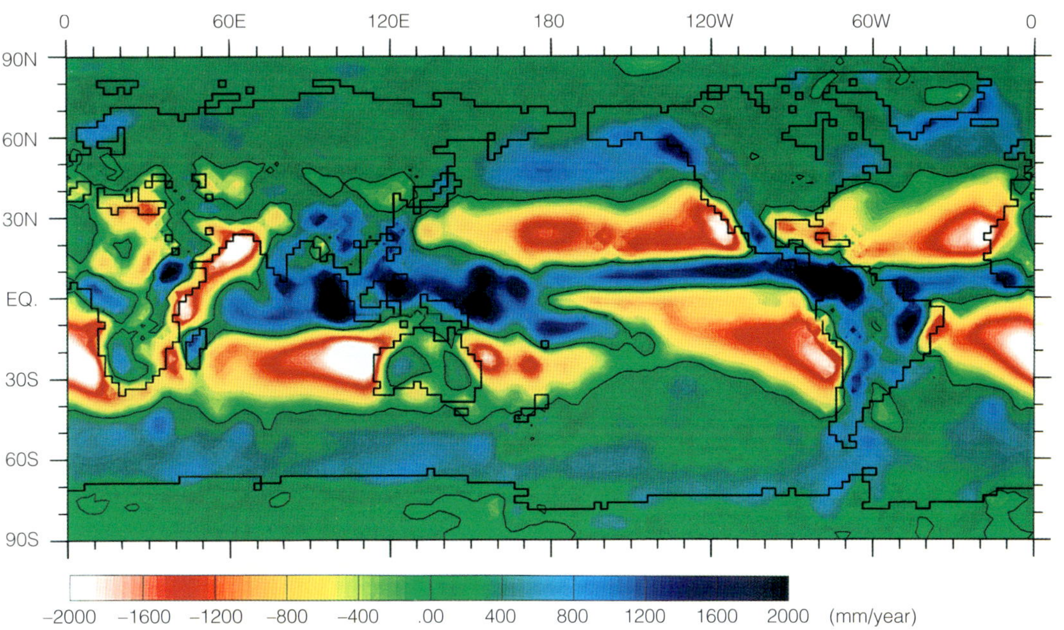

GIS application for global land use planning

In order to control global warming, C fixation such as reforestation should be encouraged. On the other hand, agricultural lands are expanding to support the growing world population. Considering both sides, an adequate land use plan must be prepared. Fig. (a) shows the suitability of land for forest conservation and reforestation. The suitable land is concentrated in tropical countries. Fig. (b) shows the actual and simulated land use in 1990 and 2025, where 30% of the forest area of 1990 is estimated to have been lost by 2025.

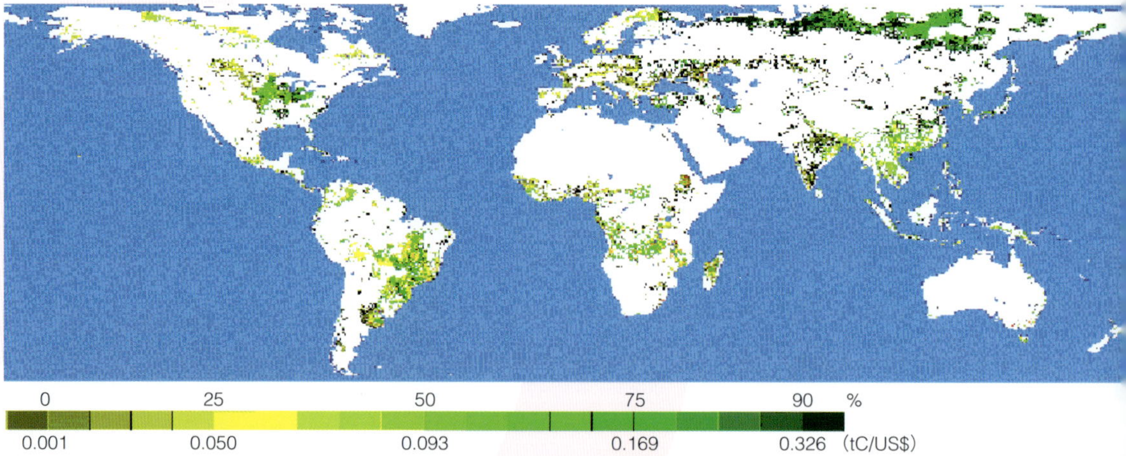

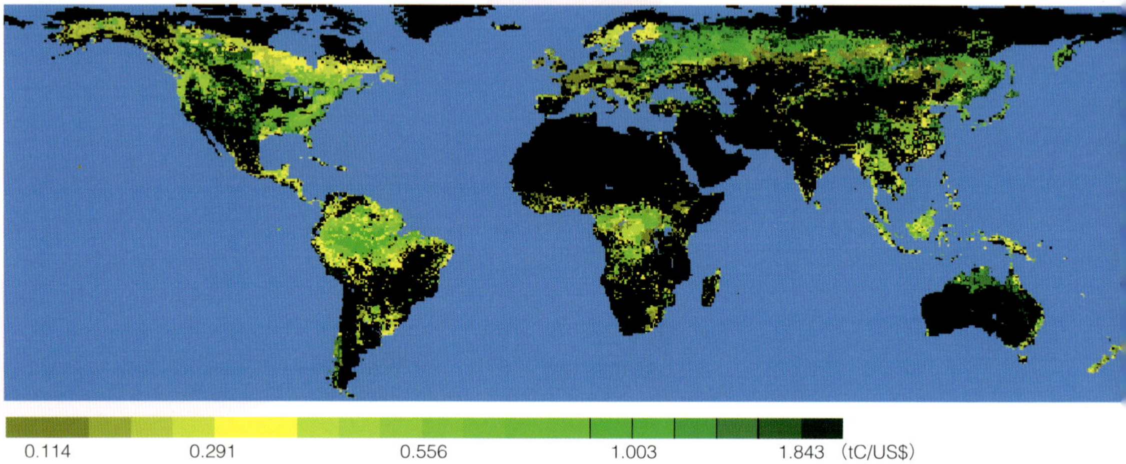

(a)

Estimation of carbon
— Content distribution in the terrestrial ecosystem

The effect of climate change on terrestrial ecosystems through the increase of atmospheric carbon dioxide has attracted much attention. For estimating these effects quantitatively, a mathematical model, which expresses the global carbon cycle is needed. For this purpose, models, which express vegetation growth and the carbon cycle in soil have been established.

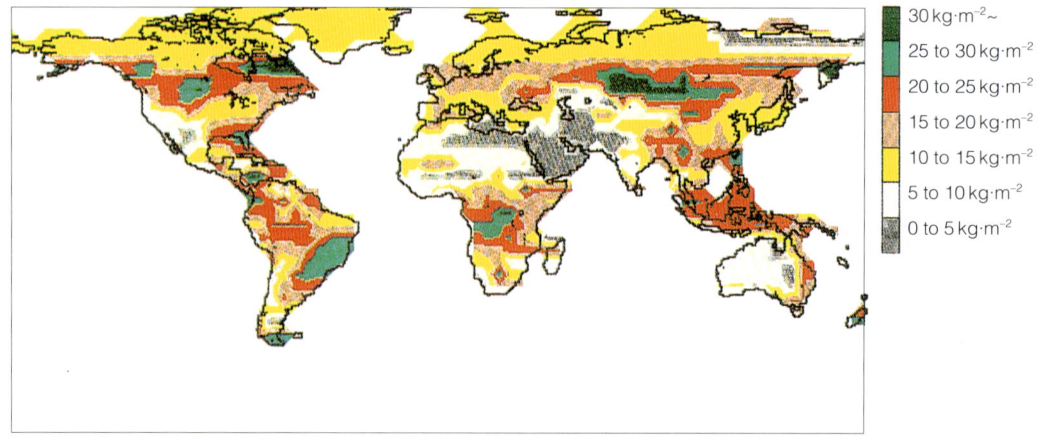

Global warming is a very serious problem, which threatens the existence of human life. In addition, the changing of forests over time shows the evidence of human activities. We will consider the problems of the global environment from the viewpoint of the earth's forests.

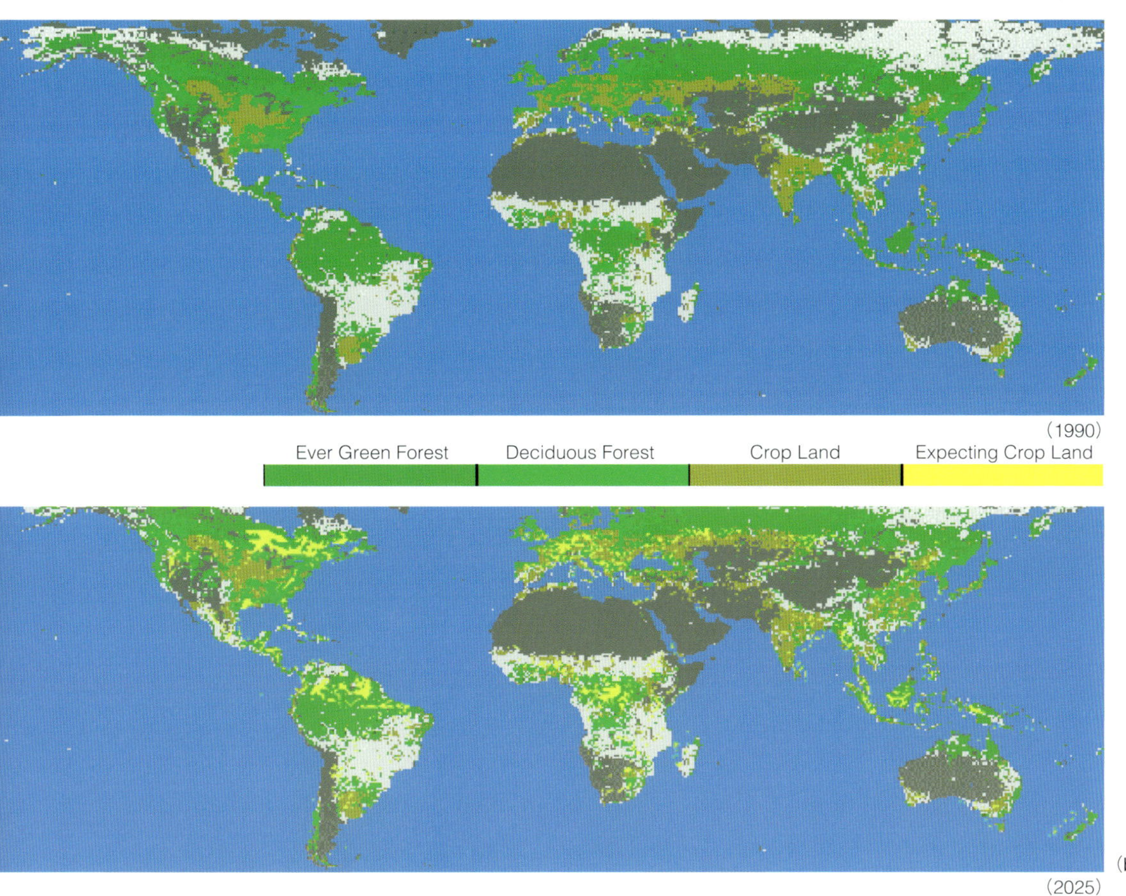

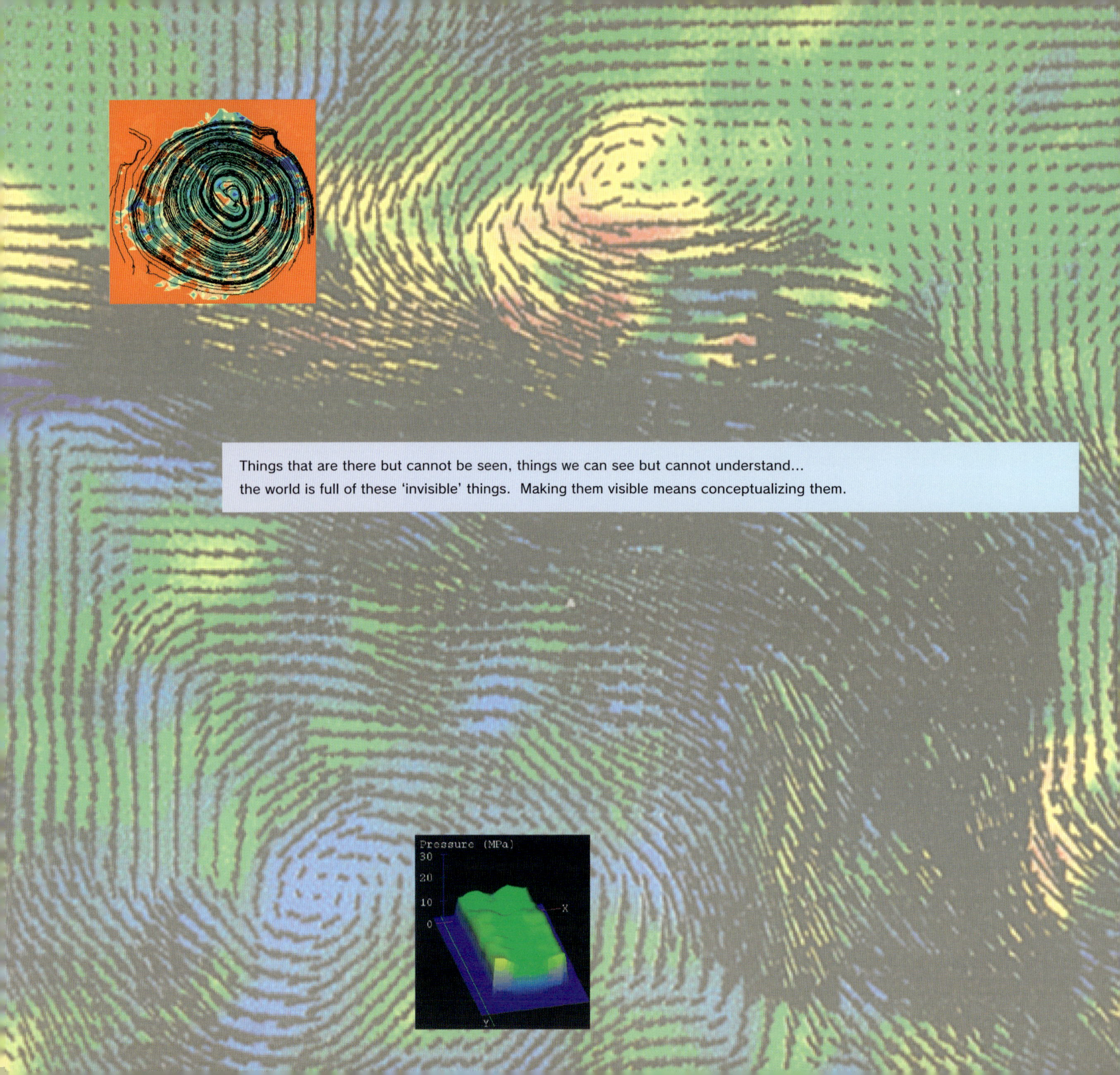

Things that are there but cannot be seen, things we can see but cannot understand…
the world is full of these 'invisible' things. Making them visible means conceptualizing them.

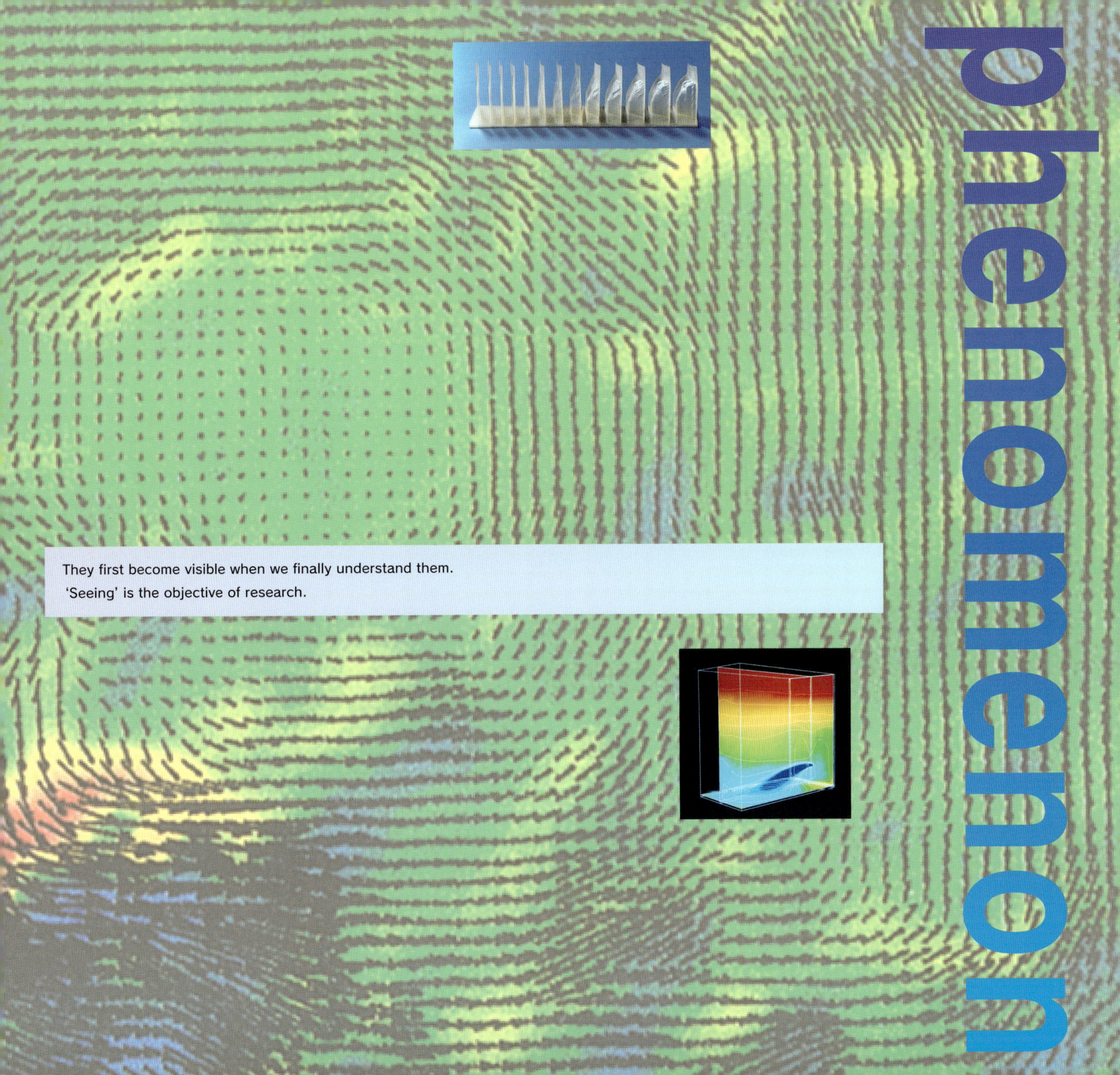

phenomenon
They first become visible when we finally understand them.
'Seeing' is the objective of research.

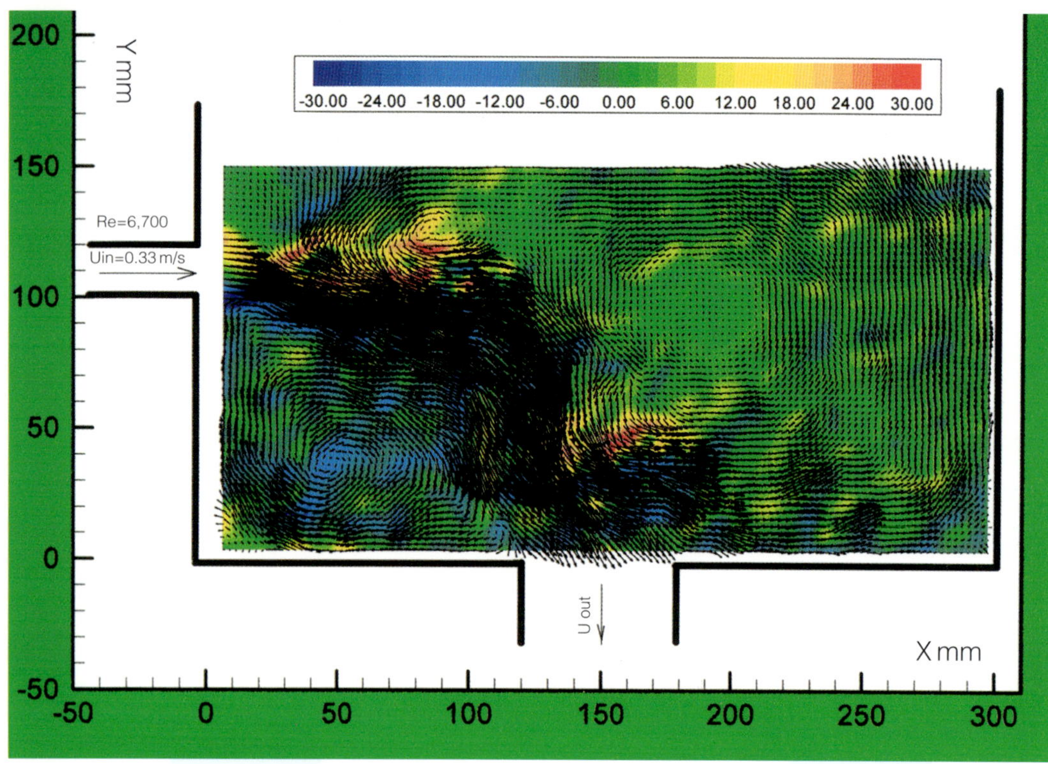

The velocity measurement in an oscillating flow field

By seeding a flow field with fine tracer particles and ignoring the relative movement of the tracer particles with the flow field, the instantaneous velocity distribution of the flow field can be measured by using an image processing technique called Particle Image Velocimetry (PIV). The figure shows a typical instantaneous velocity measurement result (about 7,500 vectors) in a self-induced sloshing flow by using the PIV technique.

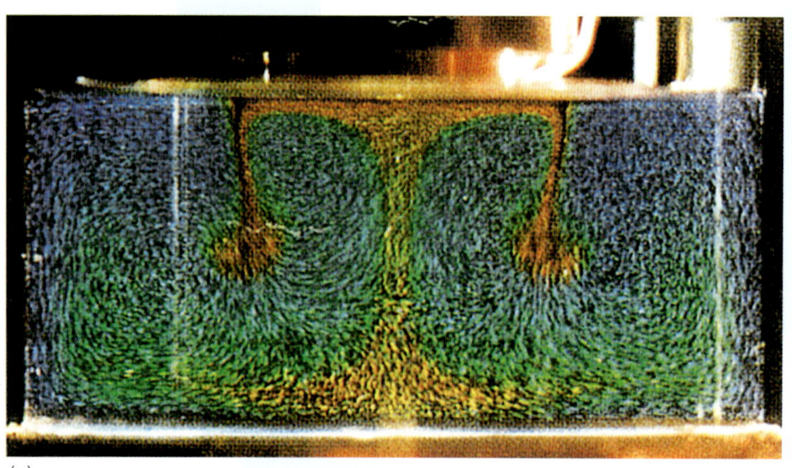

(a)

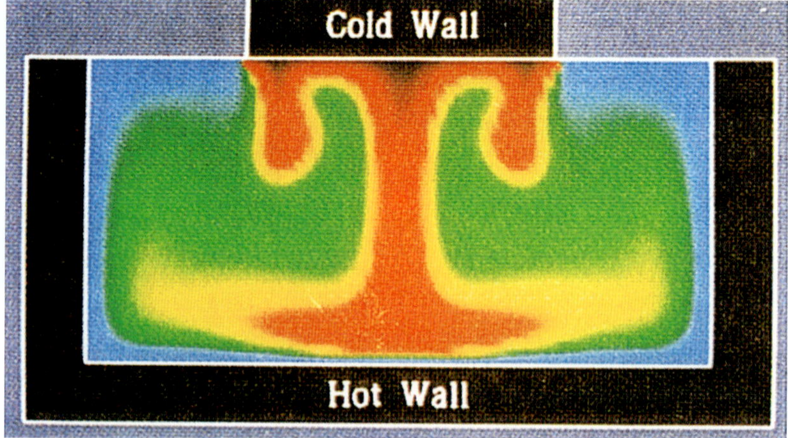

(b)

Visualization of both flow pattern and temperature distribution in a rotating cylindrical vessel

Fig. (a) shown here is a vertical view of the temperature/flow patterns using a liquid crystal encapsulated in microcapsules. Brownish parts correspond to cooler liquid while bluish parts correspond to warmer fluid. The results from the visualization were used to choose a numerical scheme to analyze the phenomena, and fig. (b) is the numerical result of temperature distribution for the situation corresponding to fig. (a).

The swirling flow in an engine cylinder

The performance of an automobile engine is related closely to fuel consumption reduction and exhaust pollutant suppression. Rarified fuel combustion was considered to be a promising solution for such problems. The figure shows a very strong swirl vortex existing in an engine cylinder according to the PIV measurement result. Such a swirling movement may result in the efficiency improvement of the rarefied fuel combustion.

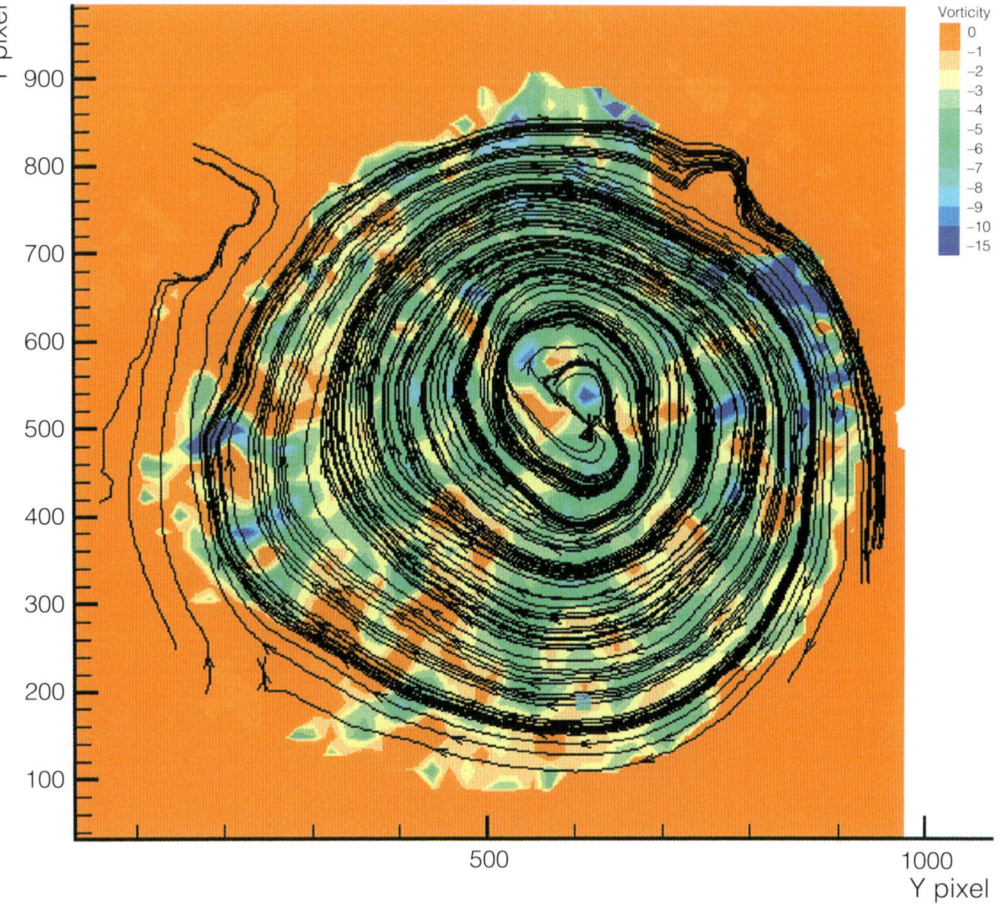

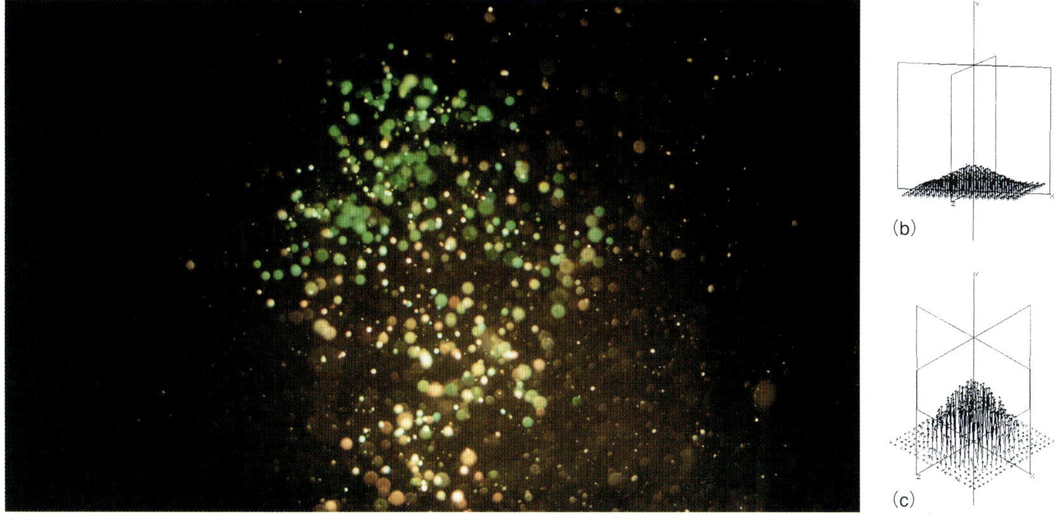

(a)

(b)

(c)

Simultaneous measurement of the temperature and velocity fields in a vertical buoyant jet flow

By using a thermo-sensitive liquid crystal tracer (fig. (a)), quantitative information such as the temperature and velocity fields of the flow field can be measured simultaneously. The right figures show the simultaneous measurement result of the three-dimensional temperature (fig. (b)) and velocity distributions (fig. (c)) in a hot buoyant jet, by using a digital color image processing technique and a stereoscopic photographing technique.

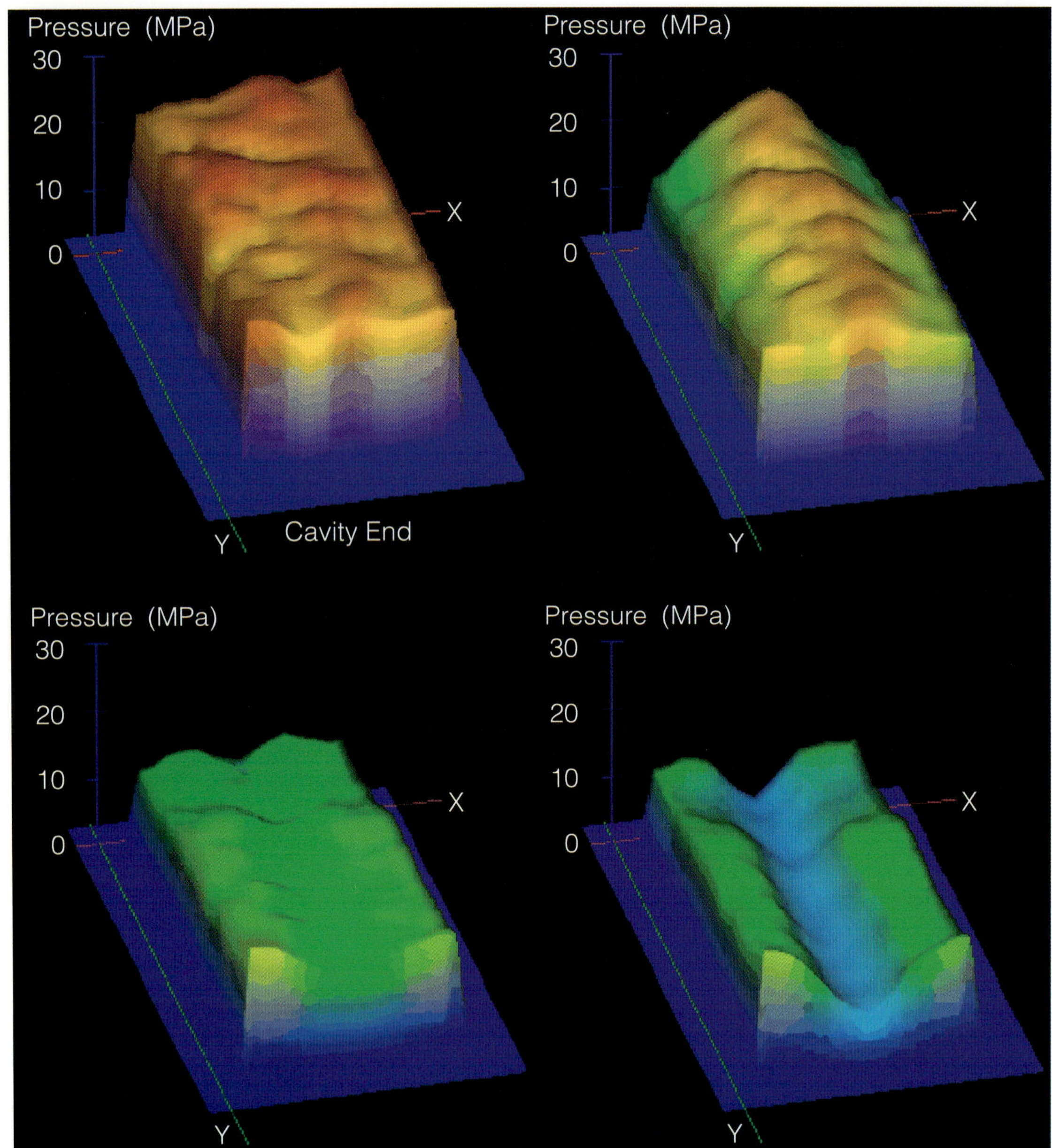

Measurement of cavity pressure distribution in injection molding

A multi-point sensing mold with an array of pressure transmission pins set on a tactile sensor enables us to measure the melt pressure distribution along the whole cavity surface. Figures show the change of pressure distribution during the pressure-molding and cooling processes in a rib-shaped cavity.

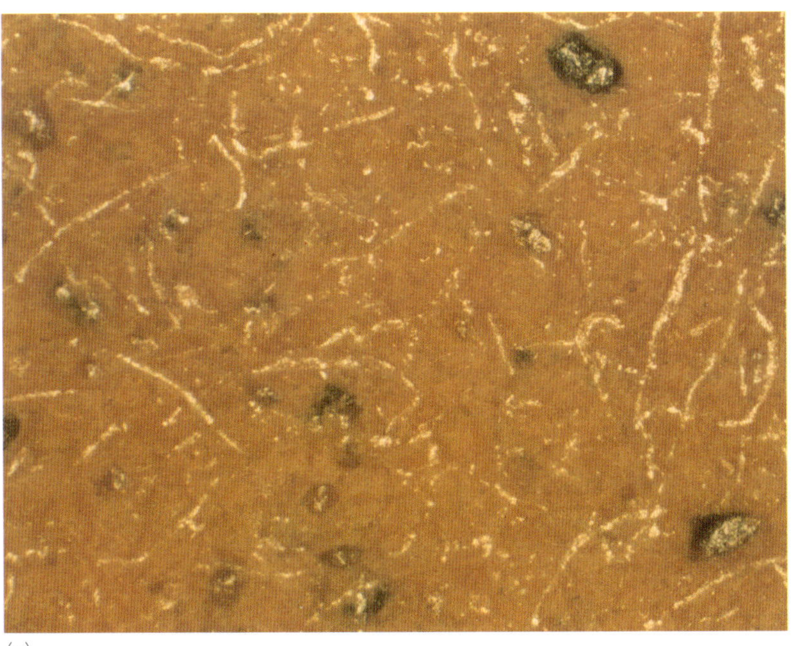

(a)

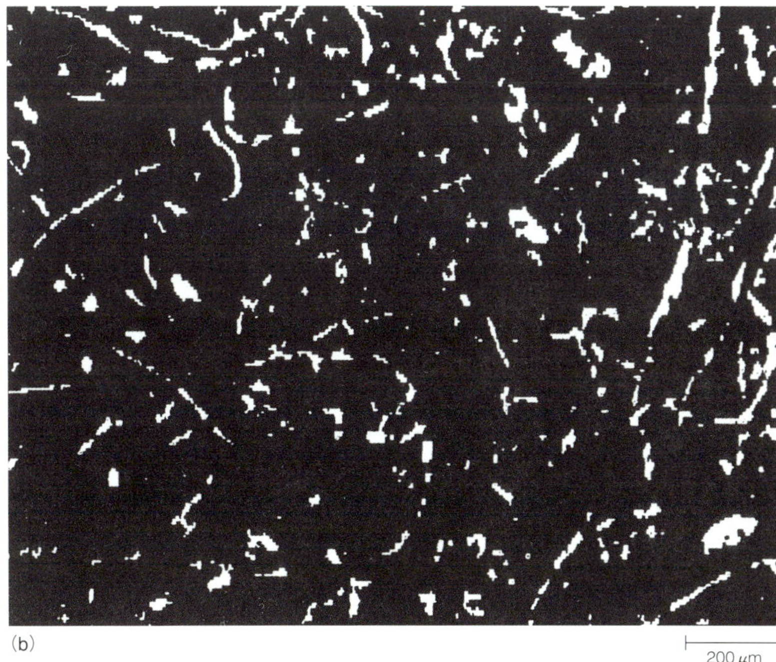

(b)

200 µm

Contact of friction material for oil-immersed clutches

Oil-immersed clutches are widely used for automatic transmission mechanisms in automobiles. For the development of friction material (fig. (a)) which has desirable friction properties to ensure a comfortable engagement, analysis is being made of its contact points formed against a glass prism, by observing the total reflection of polarized light (fig. (b)).

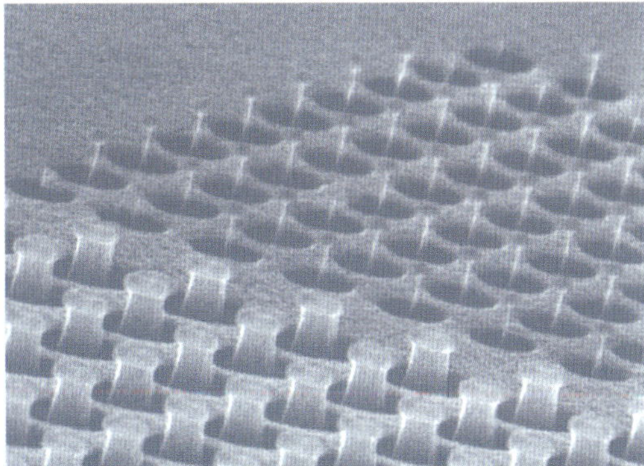

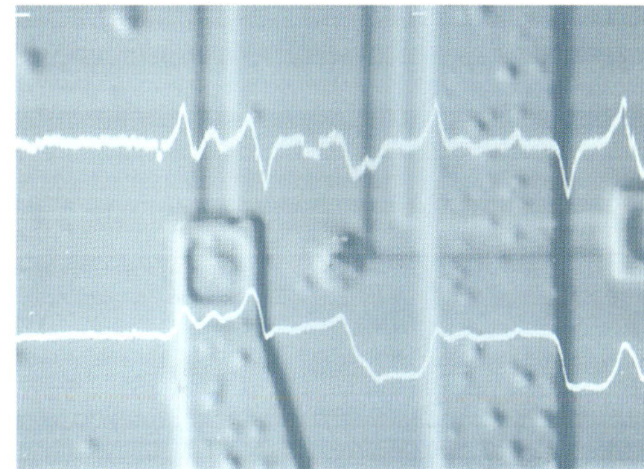

"Touching" atoms with nanometric oscillators

A nanometric mechanical oscillator has the potential of being used as a force or mass sensor at the atomic level. The figure shows an example of silicon-fabricated nanometric oscillators. The diameter of the oscillator in the background measures 100 nm.

3-D measurement of surface roughness by scanning electron microscope

The photo shows a Back-scattered Electron Image (BEI) of an IC surface by using a modified scanning electron microscope which is set at special detectors. The two white lines in the image are the line mode signal of BEI (upper line) and the topography signal (lower line). The topography signal shows the profile of the IC surface. The advantages of this method are non-contact, and great precision and speed.

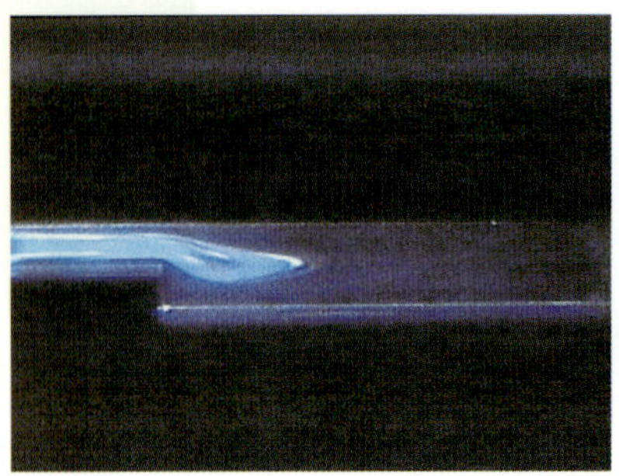 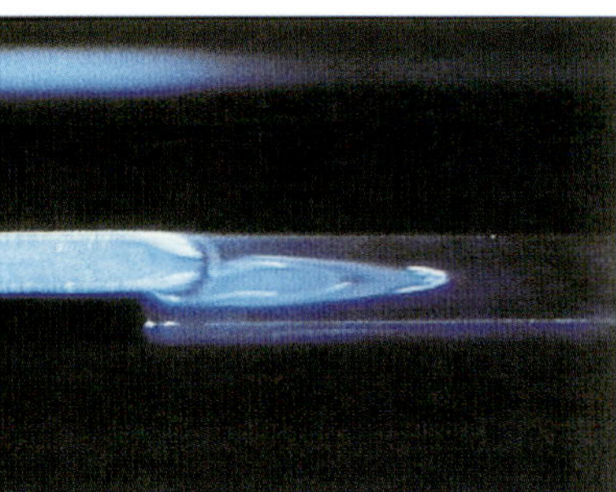 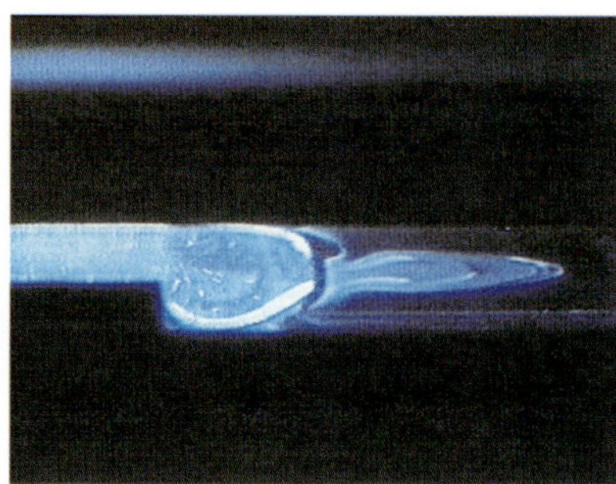 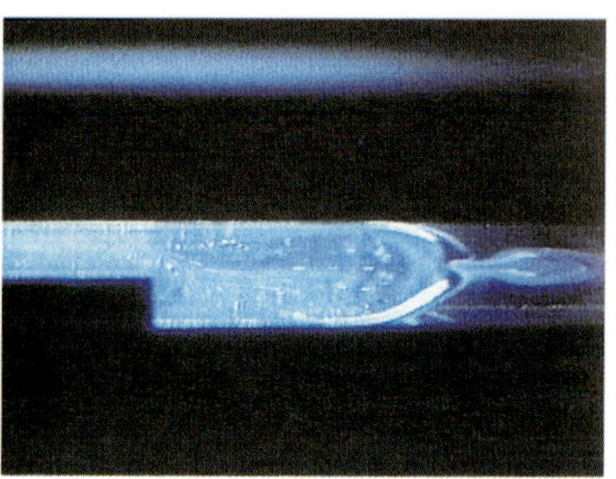

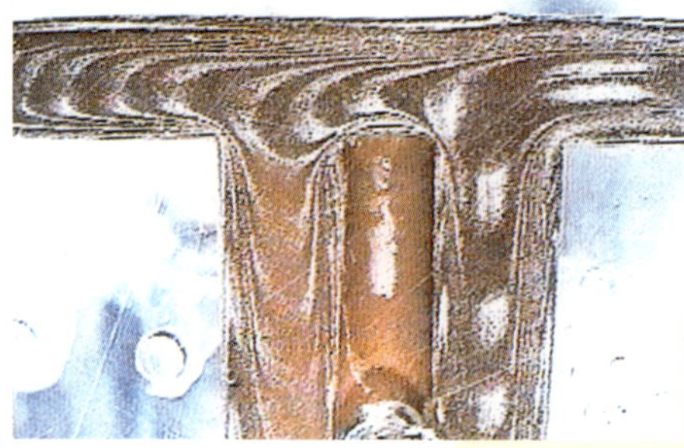

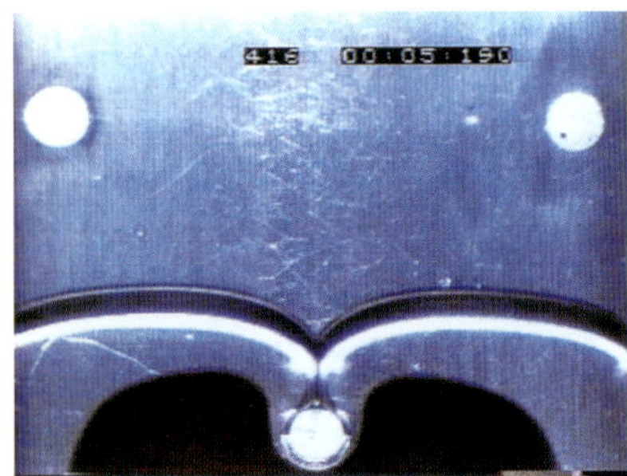 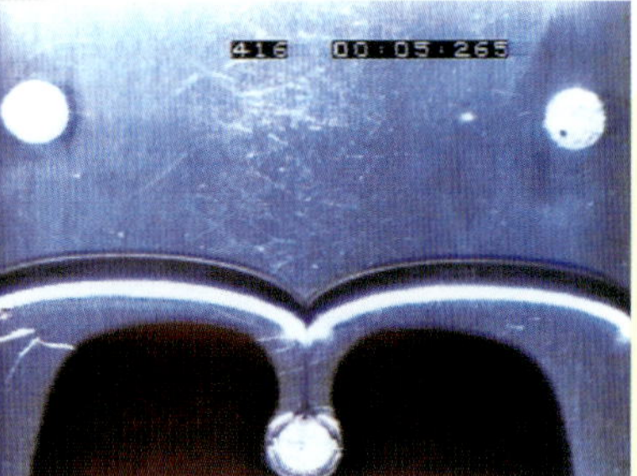 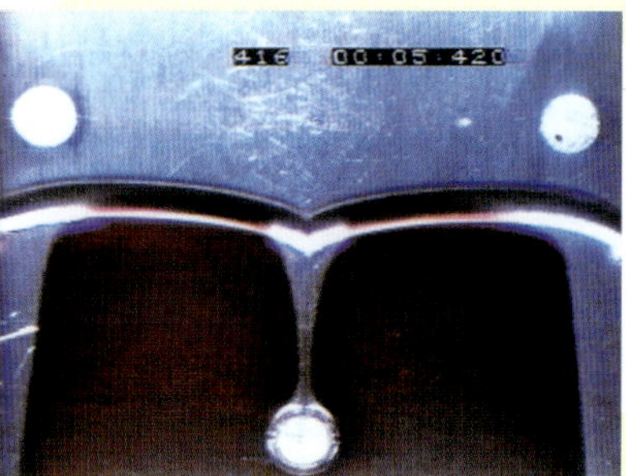 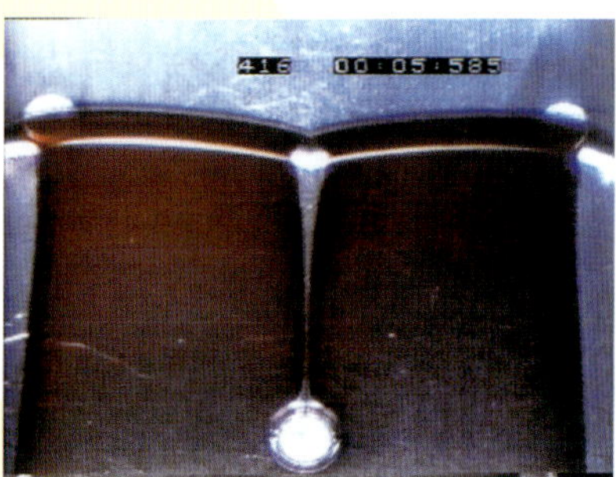

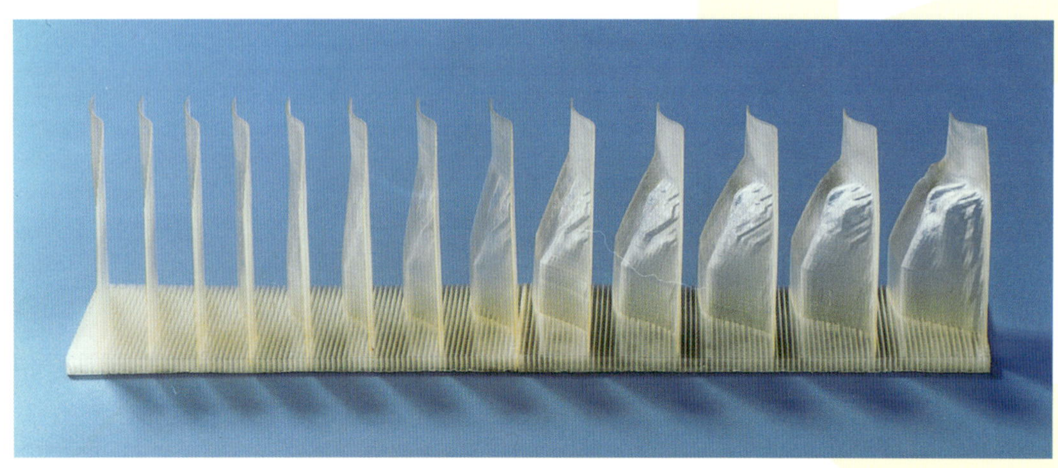

Virtual presentation of sheet metal FE simulation results by laser stereolithography

The sheet metal forming process in car body panel forming can be simulated by FE simulation. A computer simulated panel shape can be presented in its solid panel state by laser stereolithography, and we can touch the surface shape and its wrinkling with our fingers.

Visualization analyses of injection molding phenomena

In injection molding of plastics, molding equipment such as the heating cylinder and mold are fabricated from solid steel ; in effect these are like "black boxes" that prevent the complex internal phenomena from being easily elucidated. Glass-inserted molds and heating cylinders enable us to dynamically visualize various aspects of many unknown worlds.

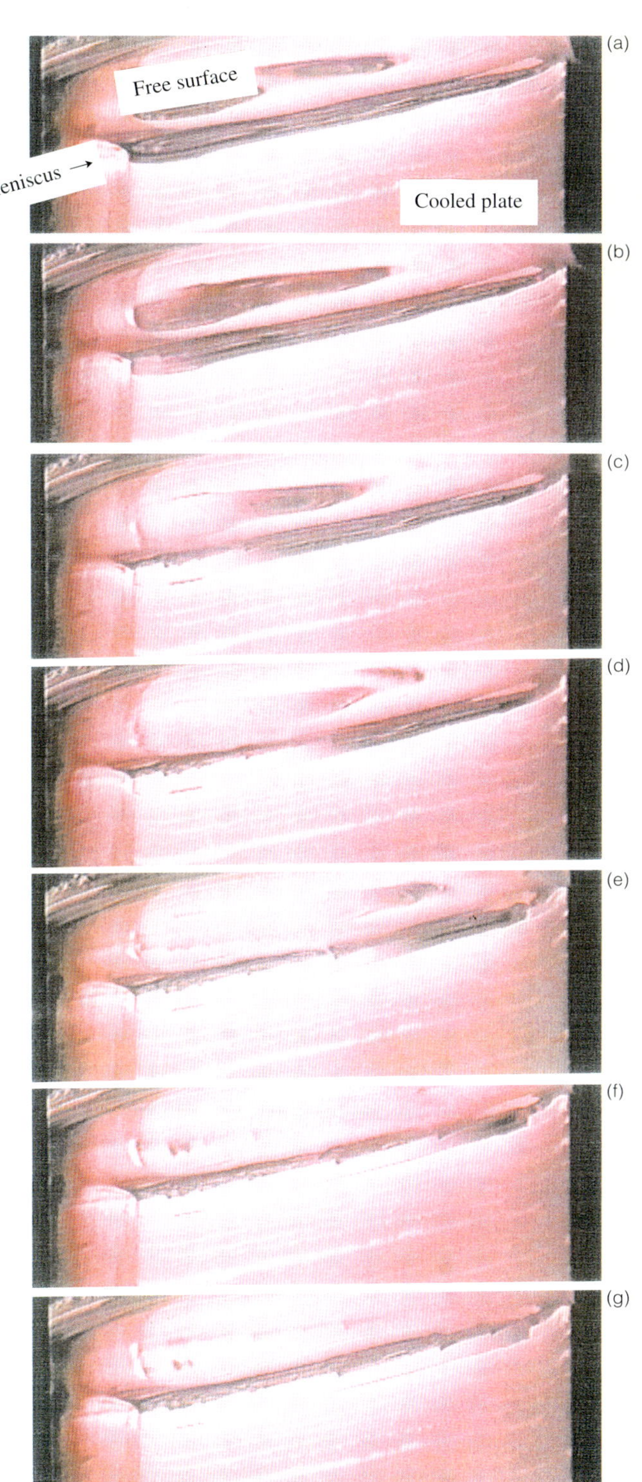

Visualization of unstable behavior of contact lines accompanied with solidification

The figures shown here are a series of front views of a chilled copper plate dipped into a pool of liquid paraffin. White parts correspond to solidified shells while brownish parts correspond to bare copper surfaces. A new cyclic phenomenon was found by the visualization, consisting of a local collapse of the meniscus, and its horizontal propagation and re-establishment.

Seeing and Making Air Currents complex phenomena around us

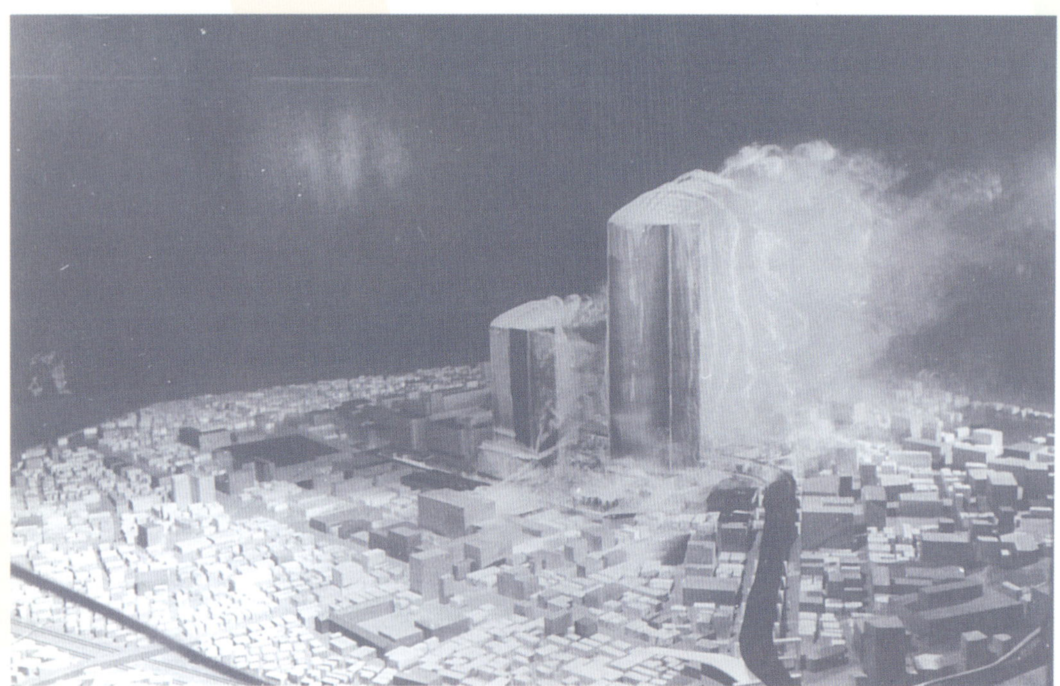

Flow visualization around high-rise building

High-rise buildings often change the wind environments at the pedestrian level greatly. Strong winds caused by them often bother pedestrians. It is therefore necessary to estimate wind effects around them before their construction. One of the reliable prediction methods is a model test in a wind tunnel. The picture shows a visualization of the wind-flow around a high-rise building model in a wind tunnel. The full-scale building is 250 m high. A 1:750 scale model was used in the wind tunnel test. As a smoke material for visualizing the flow, titanium tetrachloride was coated on the surface of the building model. The titanium tetrachloride interacts with moisture in the air and makes white smoke. This smoke can be used as a tracer for the wind-flow visualization. The vortex shedding from the top and side parts of the building can be observed in the picture.

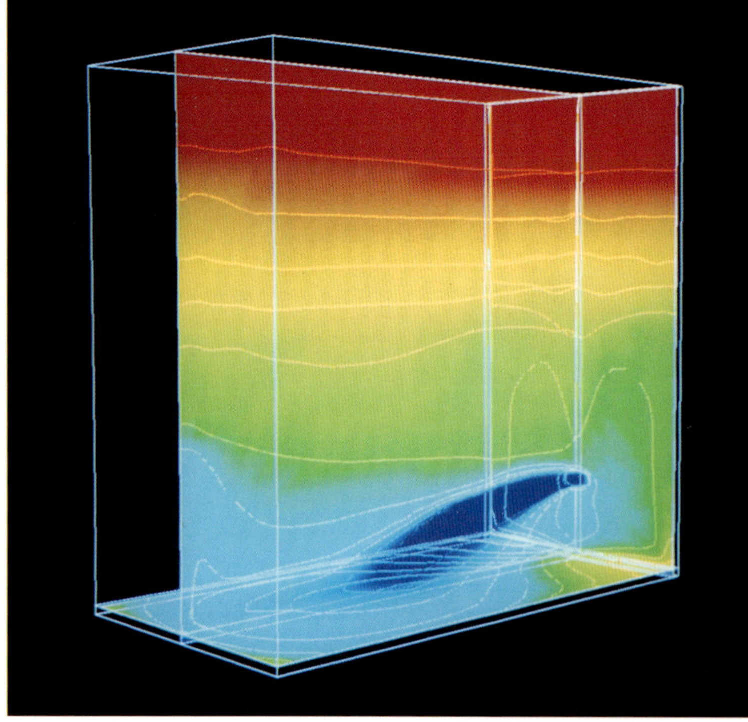

Prediction of thermal environment by using numerical simulation

Numerical simulation is used to predict the thermal environment in a building and over a city area. The picture shows the flow and temperature patterns inside an atrium by using a numerical simulation method. In the picture, the lower section region is cooled down by the cold air of Heating, Ventilation and Air-Conditioning (HVAC) and the hot air stagnates in the higher section area.

Flow analysis around 2-D cubic cylinder by using LES

An irregular, chaotic, and unpredictable motion within a flow is called a turbulent flow. By contrast, a smooth and steady flow is a laminar flow. Turbulent flows have a larger dissipation rate than laminar flows. A better understanding of the characteristics of turbulent flows is necessary in order to control wind environments around buildings. A simulation result by using Large Eddy Simulation (LES) is depicted in the figure.

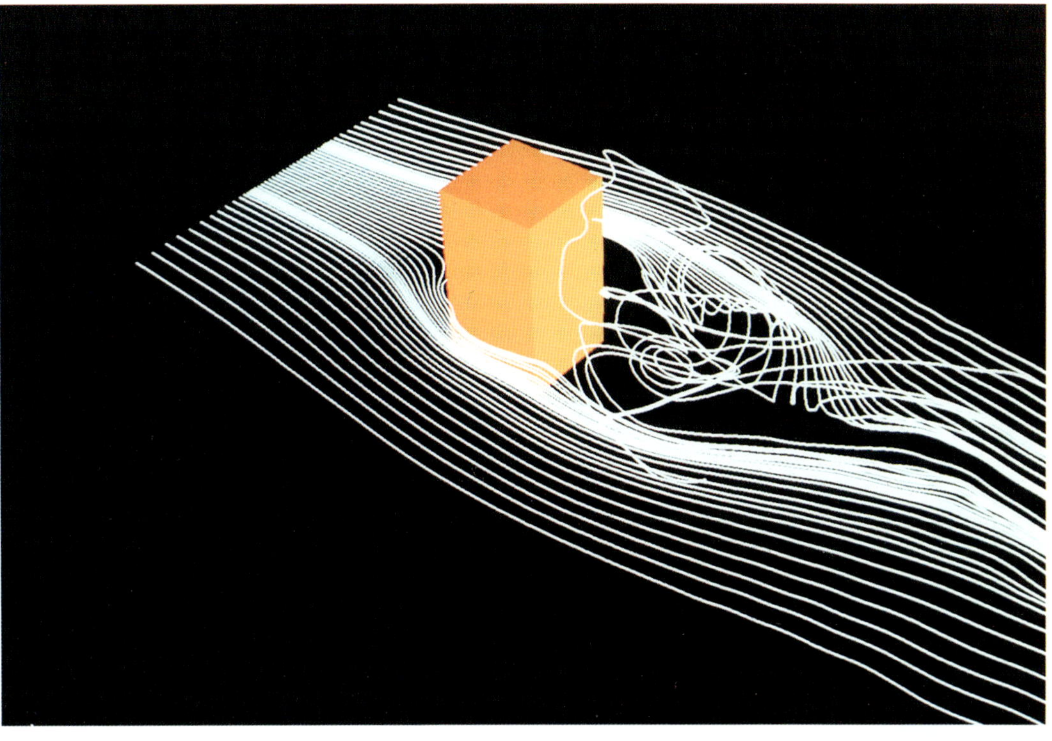

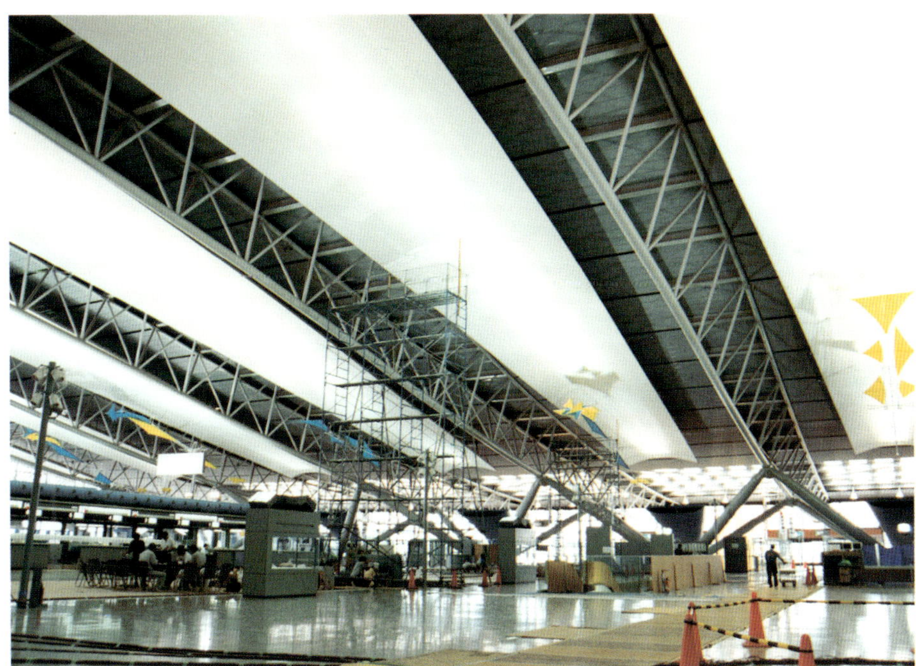

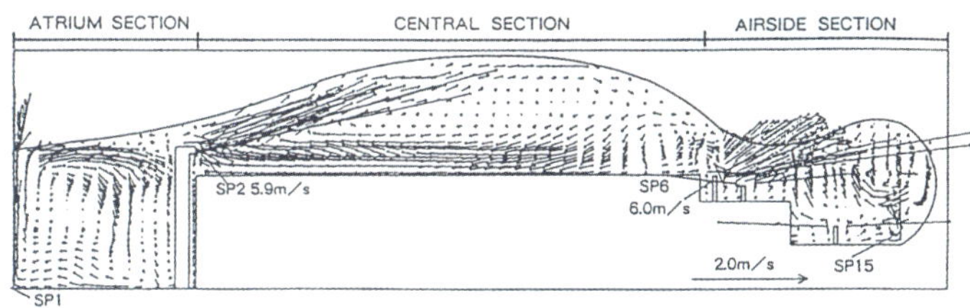

Thermal environment of large-space building

Recently, many large-space structures (e.g., indoor gymnasiums, theatres, airport terminals, etc.) have been built. The prediction for the distribution of air velocity and temperature is critical when an effective Heating, Ventilation and Air-Conditioning (HVAC) system is designed for such structures. The air velocity and temperature fields are not uniform and their distribution can be easily produced because of the size of the structures. Usually, the results obtained from numerical simulations and model tests are used to design HVAC systems for such buildings. Field-site measurements are also used as feedback to improve the next design purpose.

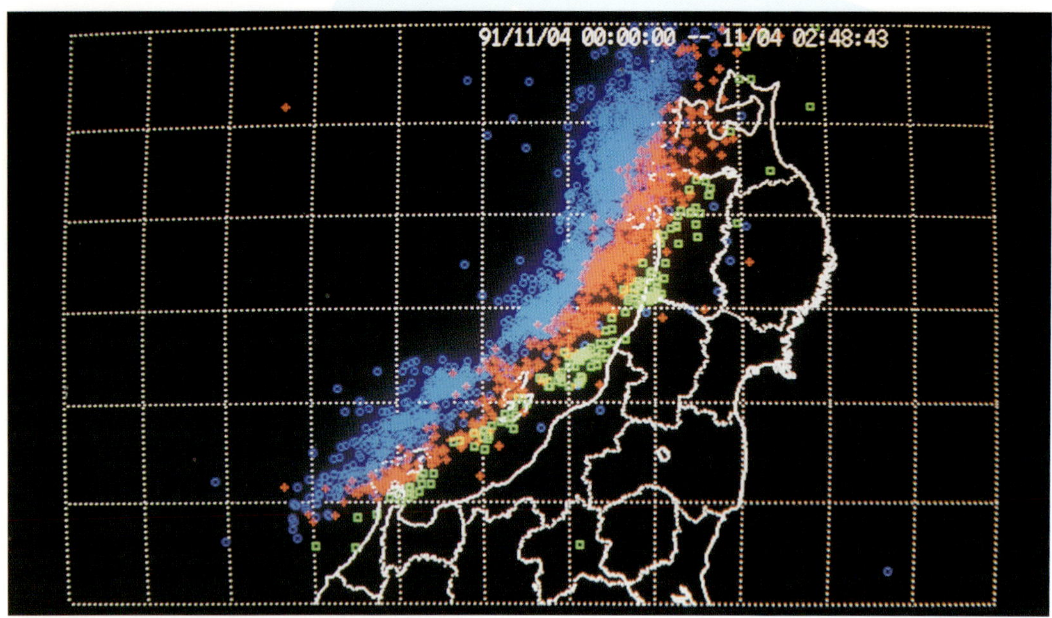

Location of lightning

Lightning discharges in a wide area are located by observing the associated electromagnetic pulses simultaneously at several receivers. The four main islands of Japan are now entirely covered by a number of such systems. The figure shows observed lightning activity in 3 hours accompanying a cold front moving from the left to the right. The color is changed every one hour.

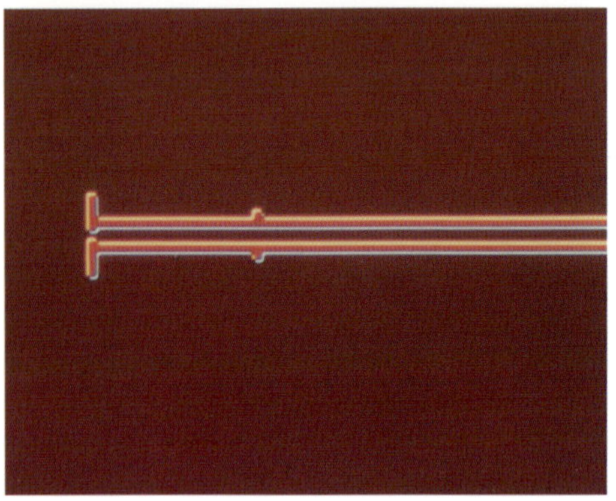

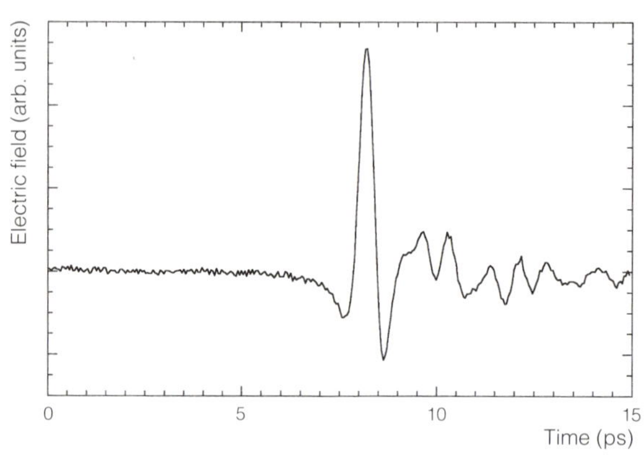

Generation and detection of terahertz electromagnetic wave by using ultrafast antenna

The THz frequency range is situated in the gap between the frequency ranges covered by conventional electronic and optical devices. However, recent developments in semiconductor and laser technologies are gradually filling this terahertz (THz) frequency gap. The photo shows an ultrafast antenna with a dimension of 1/2 of a human hair fabricated on a GaAs film grown at low temperatures (photoconductive antenna). By irradiating the gap of the antenna with femtosecond laser pulses, the generation and detection of THz radiation has become possible (diagram). The photoconducting ultrafast antenna is also providing a new tool for investigating the dynamics of ultrafast phenomena in solids.

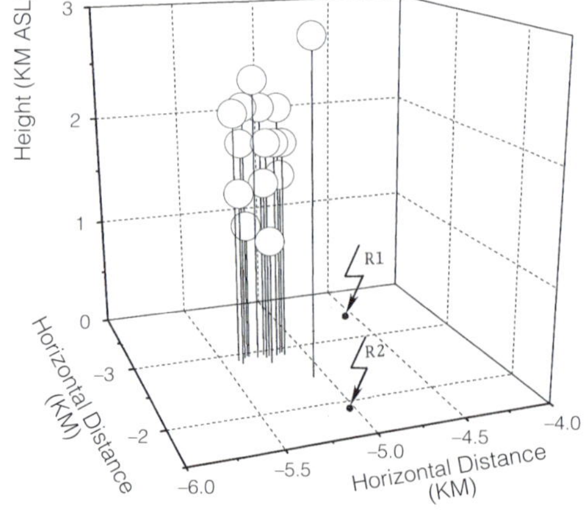

3-D Location of radiation sources asociated with lightning discharges

A lightning flash is a cluster of numerous small discharges mostly within thunderclouds, and their location is closely related to the characteristics of lightning. The figure shows the sources of discharges, three-dimensionally located from the times-of-arrival of the associated electromagnetic pulses at multiple stations, which occurred in February 1995 on the coast of the Sea of Japan. They preceded return strokes R1 and R2, and the altitudes were much lower than in summer.

Visualization of ultrafast motion of electrons by time-domain terahertz spectroscopy

It is becoming very important to understand the dynamics of electrons in modern ultrafast electron devices. We have succeeded in visualizing electron motion with 100 femtosecond time resolution, through detecting weak terahertz (THz) electromagnetic radiation by a photoconductive dipole antenna in a time domain. The diagram shows a temporal trace of THz radiation emitted by the back-and-forth tunneling motion of electrons in coupled quantum wells. Time-domain THz spectroscopy is a powerful tool for clarifying real-time motions of electrons.

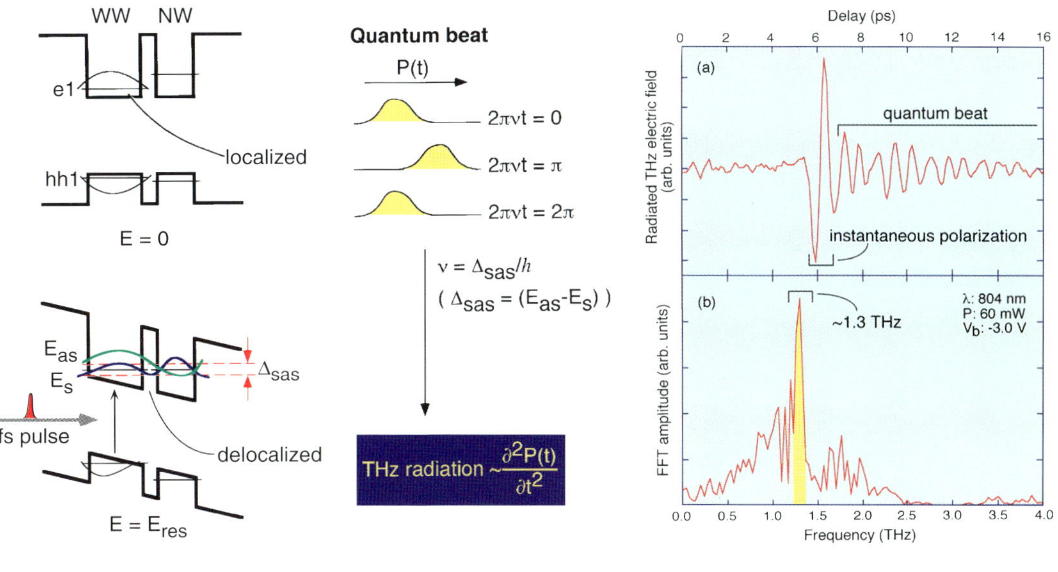

Soliton logic circuit

The fiber-optic soliton is considered to be promising for the long-haul optical communication system. The soliton can also provide a kind of logic circuit element. This logic circuit consists of an asymmetrical non-linear fiber-optic coupler. This gives a new logical AND and OR circuit under certain conditions. This logic circuit can be realized in a long transmission fiber. This soliton logic circuit is proposed and analyzed, and may contribute to the development of solitonics technology.

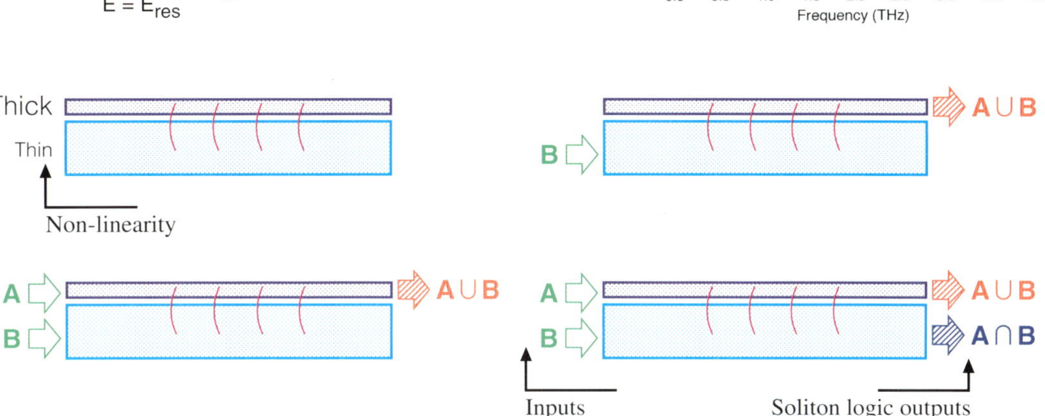

Research on tropical lightning

Observation of lightning in Indonesia has been carried out as a joint research with the Bandung Institute of Technology, Bandung. A lightning location system comprising four stations covered the island of Java, and operated during 1994-1996. The figure shows an example of the distribution of lightning flashes in the rainy season. Lightning activity is almost restricted to the island and off the coast.

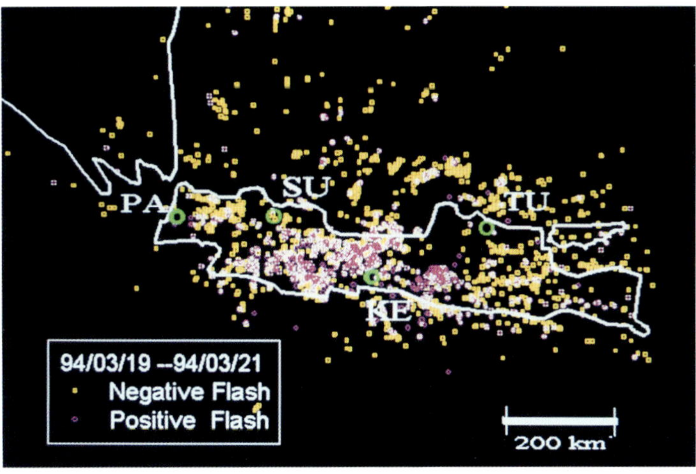

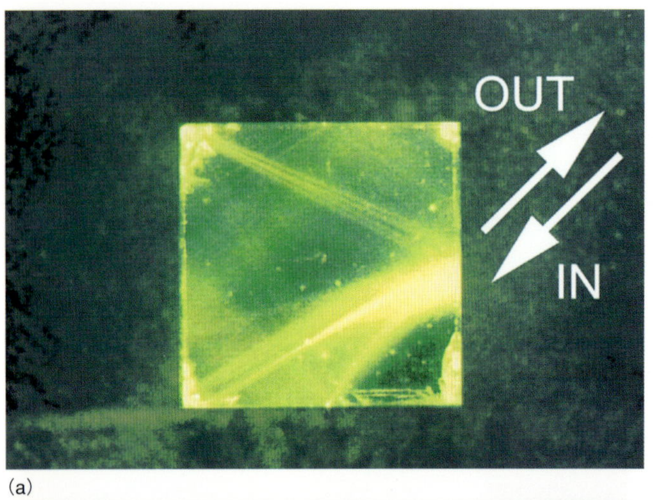

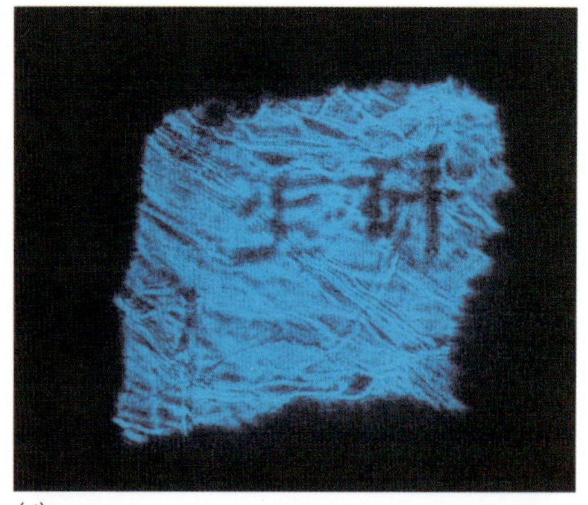

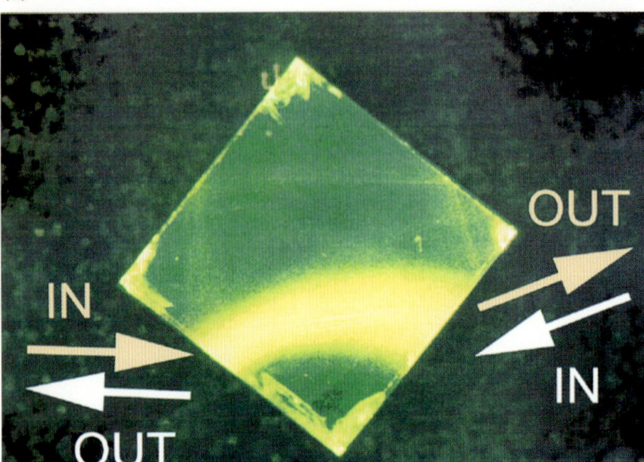

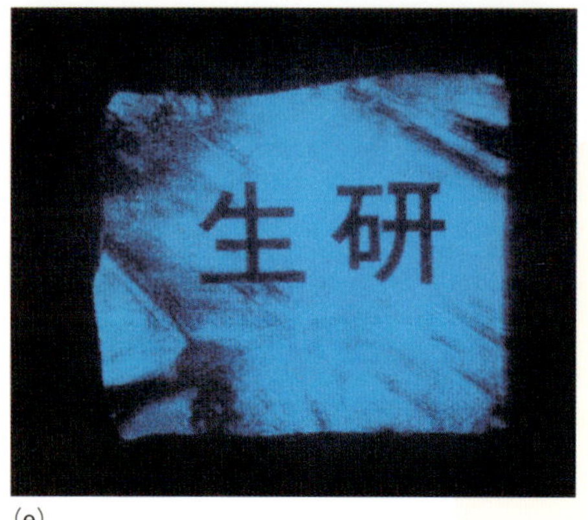

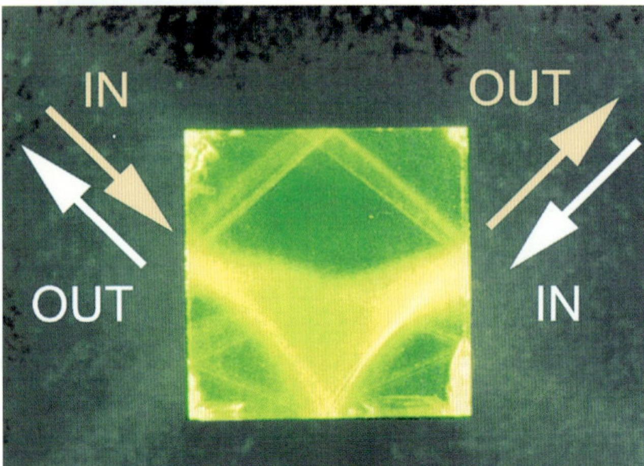

Optical phase conjugate mirrors using BaTiO$_3$
Optical phase conjugate waves can be generated with astonishing ease by using a BaTiO$_3$ single crystal. We have only to input one laser beam into the crystal. The beam forms its path loop by generating small gratings inside the crystal and traces back exactly the same path (fig. (a)). We can also obtain two phase conjugate beams simultaneously with two input beams (fig. (b), (c)). These phase conjugate mirrors can recover the clear image (fig. (e)) even if it is once distorted (fig. (d)).

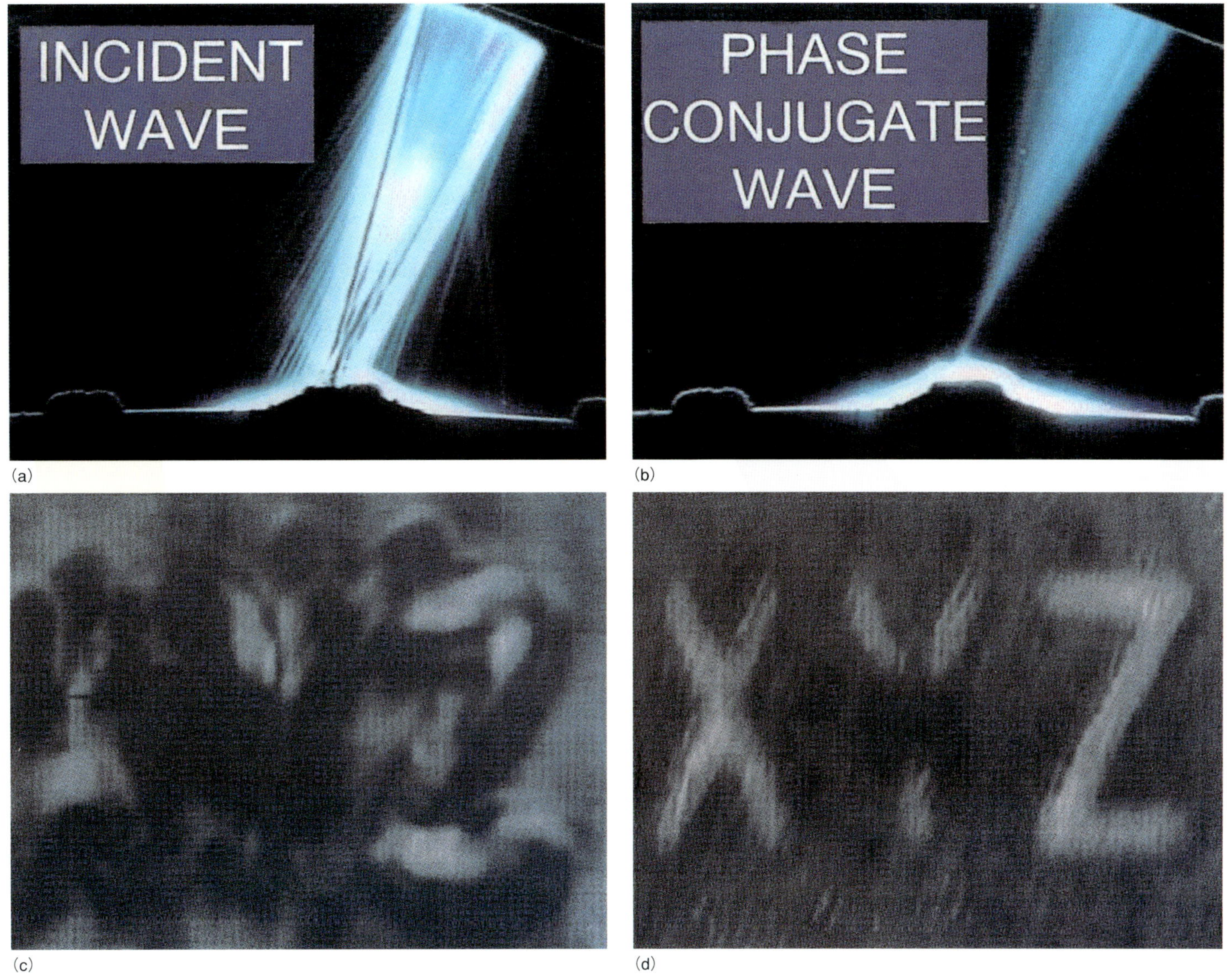

Acoustic phase conjugate waves — Generation and visualization

We developed an acoustic phase conjugate "mirror", which generates the phase conjugate wave of the incident ultrasonic wave. We can observe this process by the schlieren technique, which enables us to see ultrasonic waves directly. The incident wave converges on the mirror (fig. (a)), and then its phase conjugate wave diverges (fig. (b)). Phase conjugate waves have the property of auto-correction of the distorted wavefront, which is useful in improving the quality of the picture obtained by an ultrasonic imaging system (fig. (c), (d)).

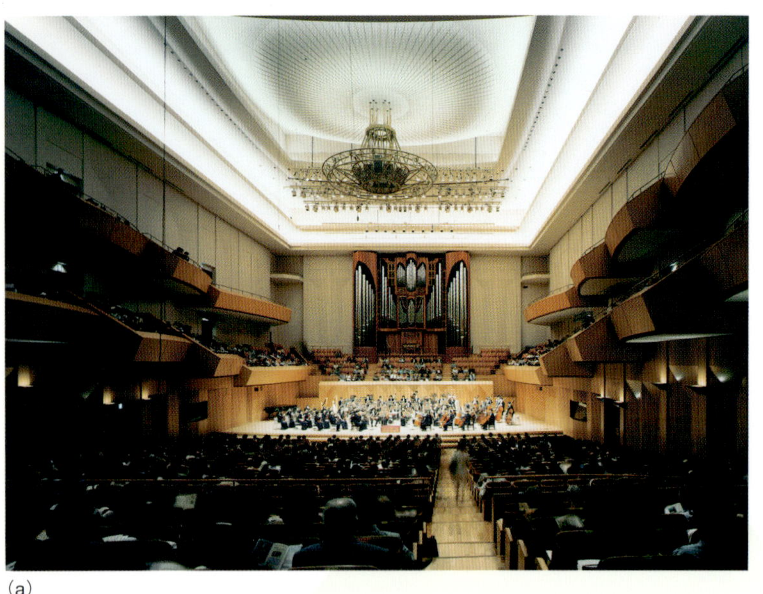

(a)

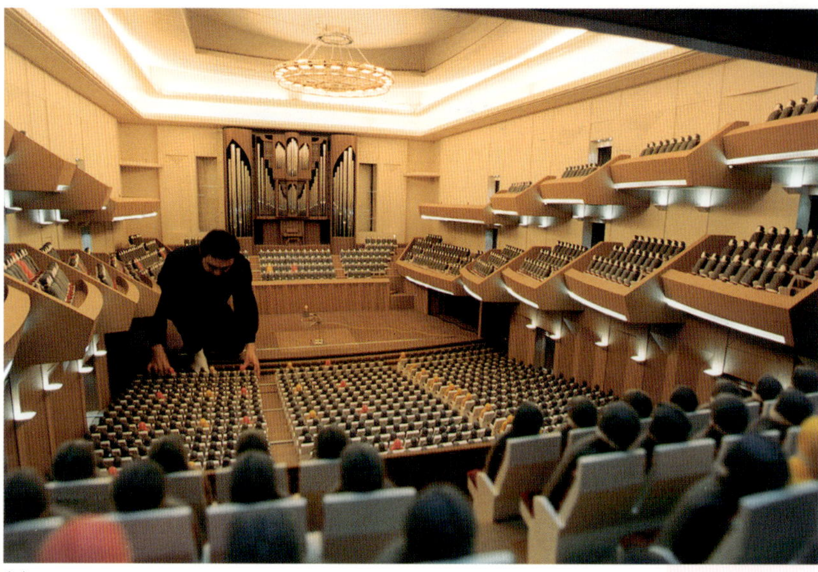

(b)

Scale model experiment of concert hall acoustics

In the design process of concert halls and opera houses, scale model experiments to predict their room acoustics are often performed by applying the Hybrid Acoustic Simulation Technique developed by I.I.S., by which audition of music played in the hall (hall sound) can be performed in addition to the measurements of acoustic parameters (photo by Tokyu Construction CO, ltd.).

(a)

(b)

Visualization of sound power flow from a musical instrument

The sound intensity measurement method is useful for the visualization of acoustic radiation characteristics from sound sources. As an example of its application, the figure shows the measurement results of sound energy flow from a violoncello (open second string D). In the left figure, the sound power is radiated uniformly from the f-hole at the fundamental frequency (147 Hz, fig. (a)), whereas in the right figure local sound absorption (sink) can be seen at the second harmonic frequency (293 Hz, fig. (b)).

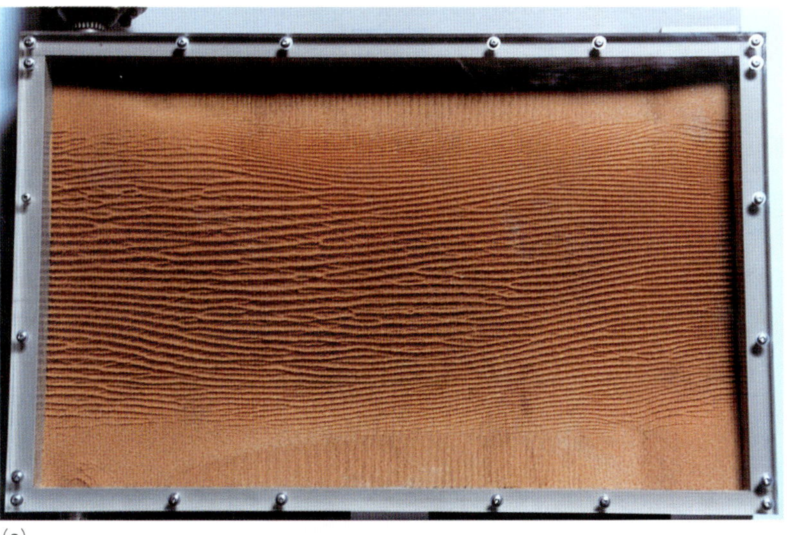

(a)

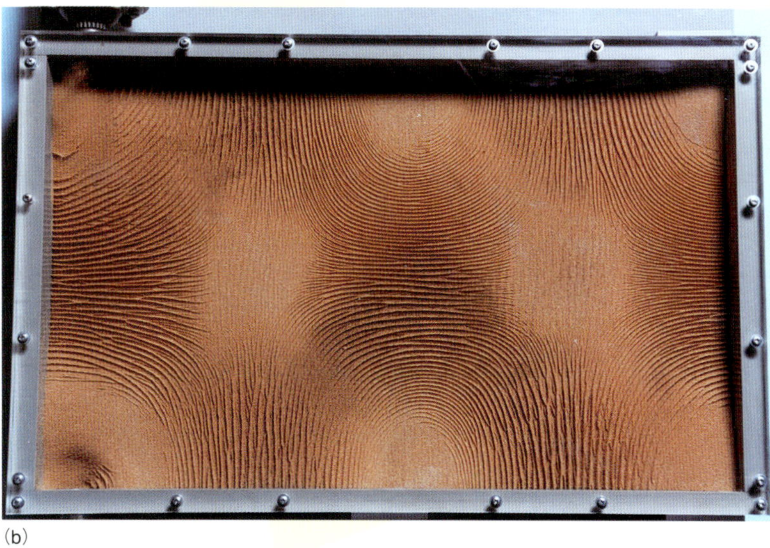

(b)

Visualization of acoustic resonance by the Kundt's experiment method

Photographs show the acoustic resonance in a 2-D room visualized by applying the Kundt's dust-tube method using cork dust as the tracer. When the sound field is excited by a sound corresponding to the resonance frequency determined by the dimension of the room, the cork dust is violently excited in the area where air particle velocity is high and the standing wave mode can be clearly observed as uniform striped patterns. Fig. (a): (1, 0) mode; fig. (b): (1, 2) mode.

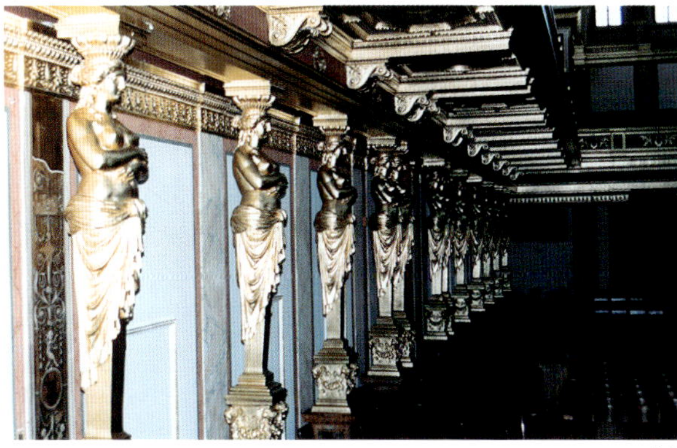

(a)

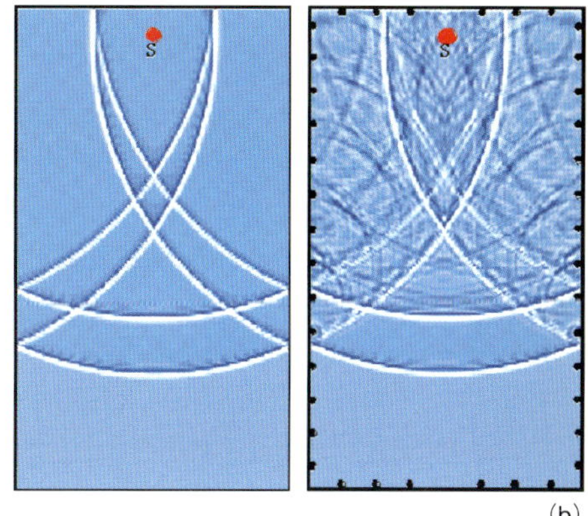

(b)

Analysis of sound diffusion by numerical simulation

The photograph shows the side wall of the Vienna Musikvereinssaal, one of the most world-famous concert halls, which has an array of columns ornamented with female statues (fig. (a)). It is believed that they make the hall acoustically excellent. In order to examine this point, numerical analysis based on FDM was performed by modeling the statues (fig. (b)). In the results, it can be clearly seen that the pulse sound radiated from the source point (S) is effectively scattered by the column array (right) compared with the case without the array (left).

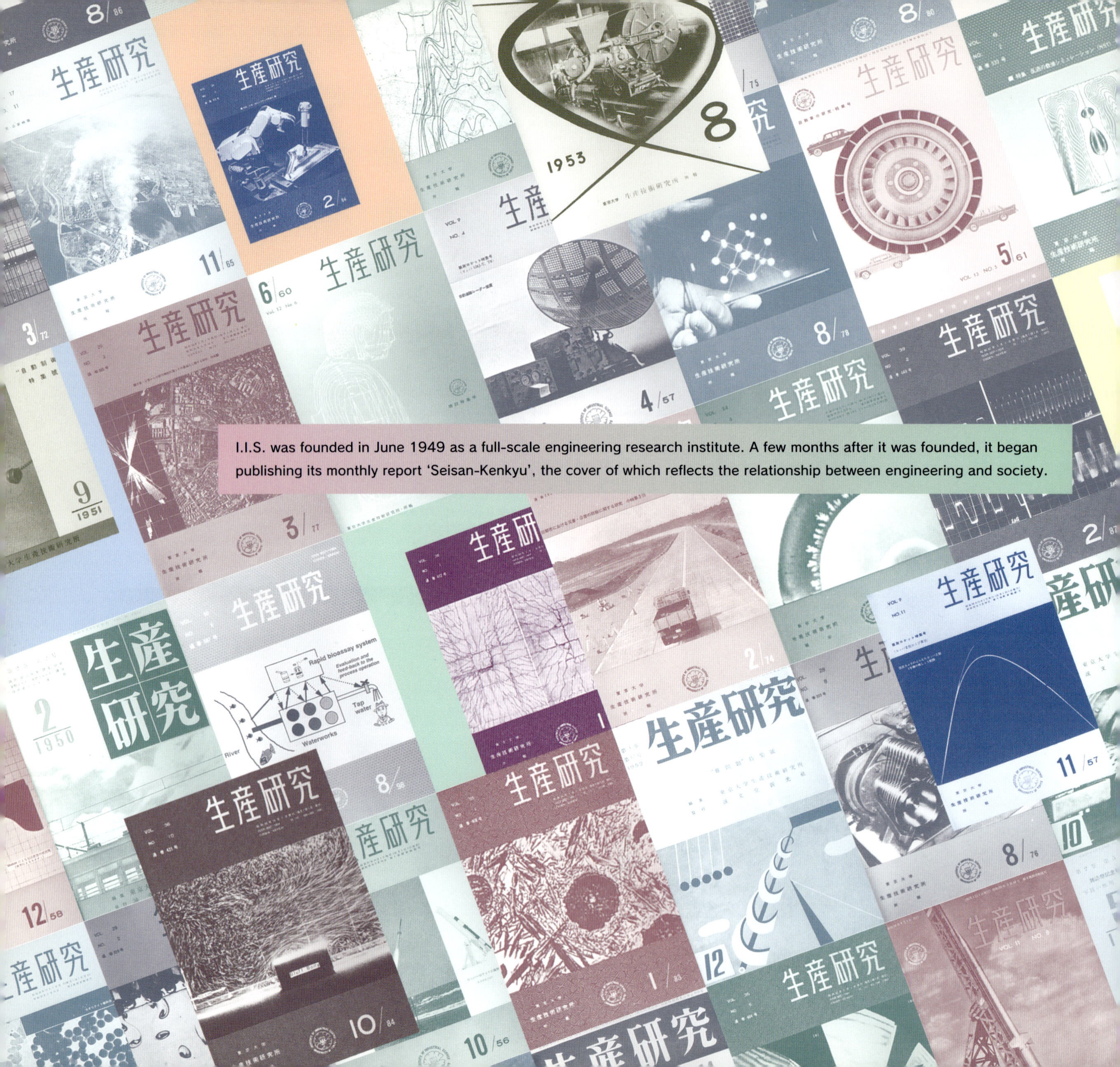

I.I.S. was founded in June 1949 as a full-scale engineering research institute. A few months after it was founded, it began publishing its monthly report 'Seisan-Kenkyu', the cover of which reflects the relationship between engineering and society.

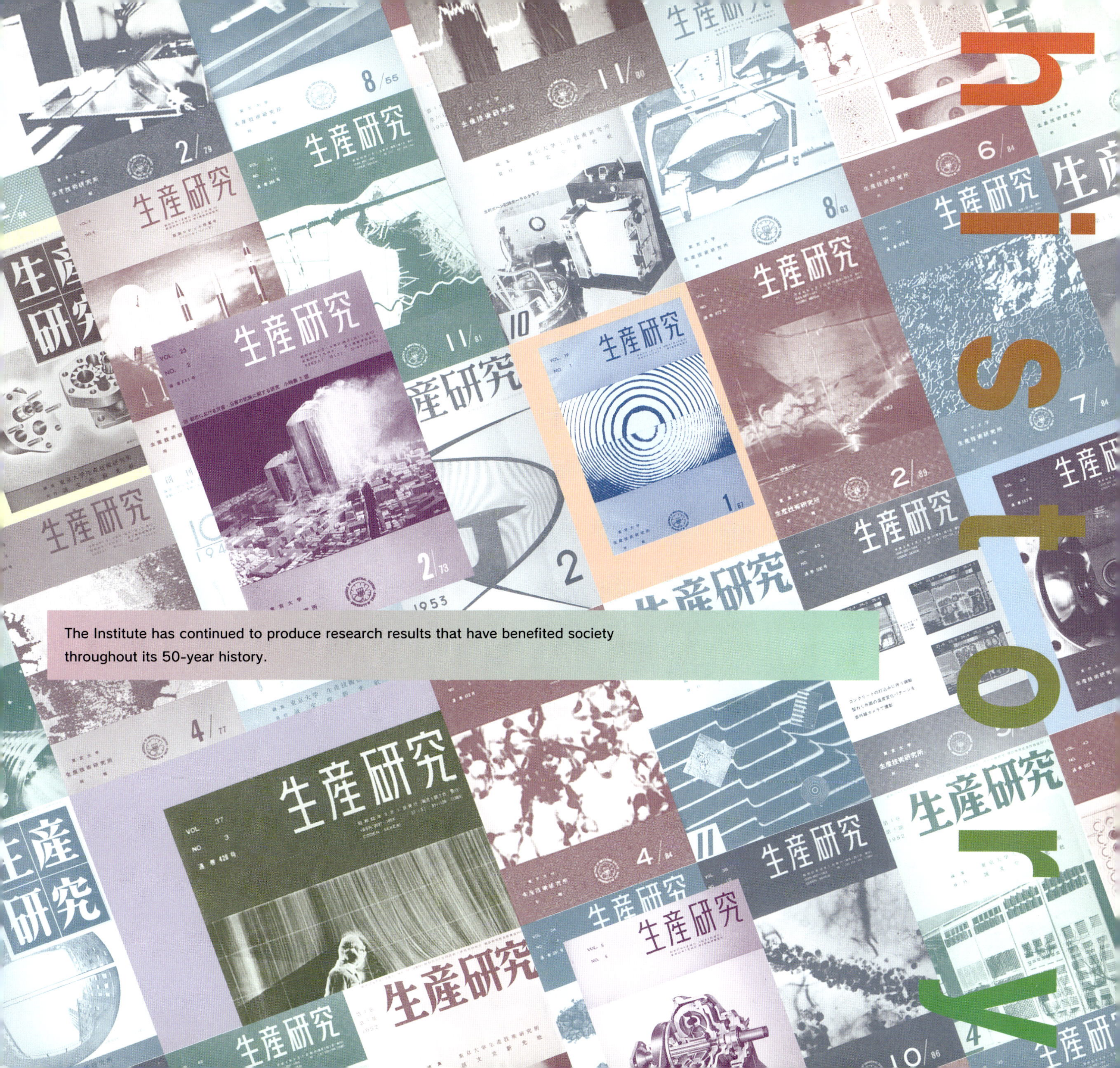

history
The Institute has continued to produce research results that have benefited society
throughout its 50-year history.

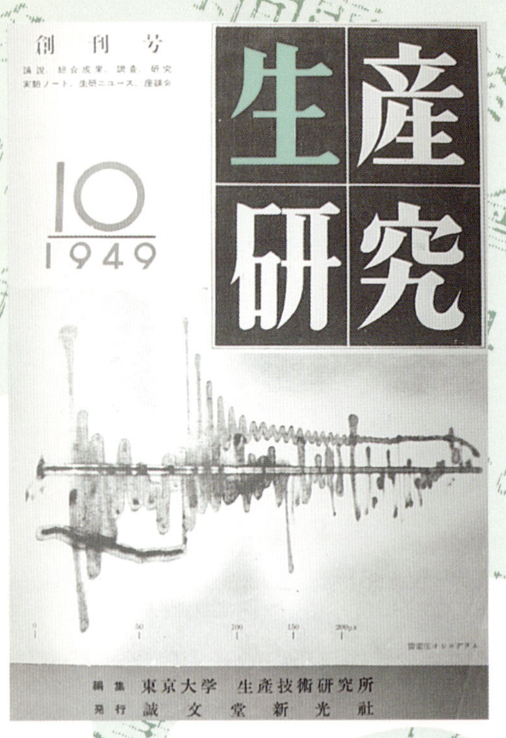
創刊号
生産研究
10
1949
編集　東京大学　生産技術研究所
発行　誠文堂新光社

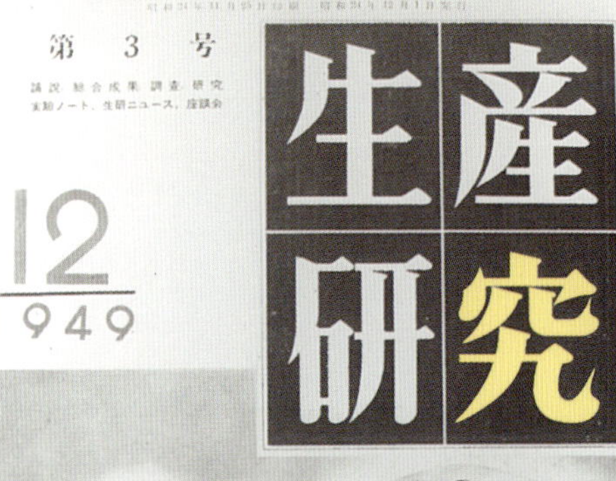

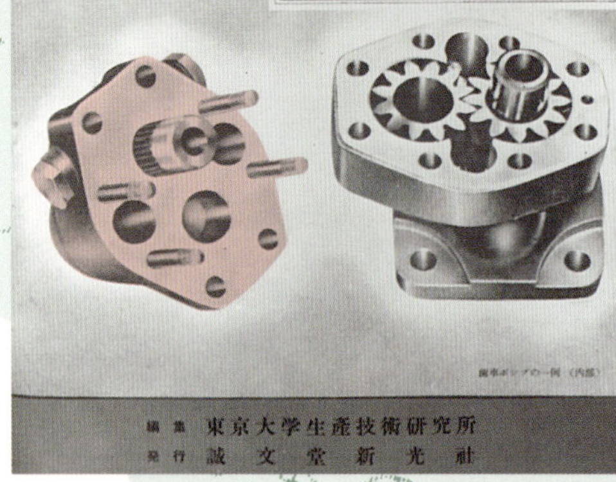
第 3 号
生産研究
12
1949
編集　東京大学生産技術研究所
発行　誠文堂新光社

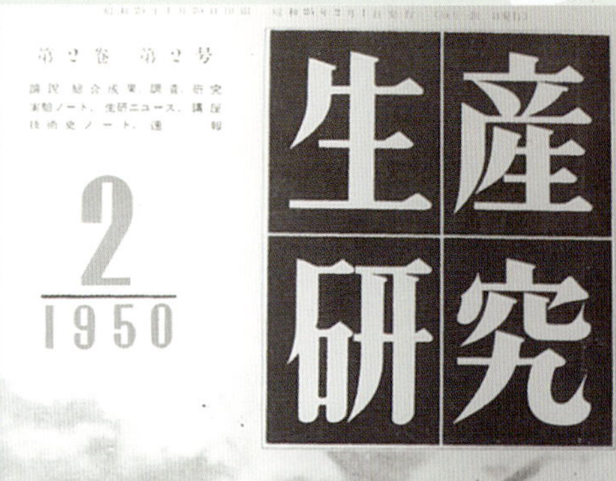

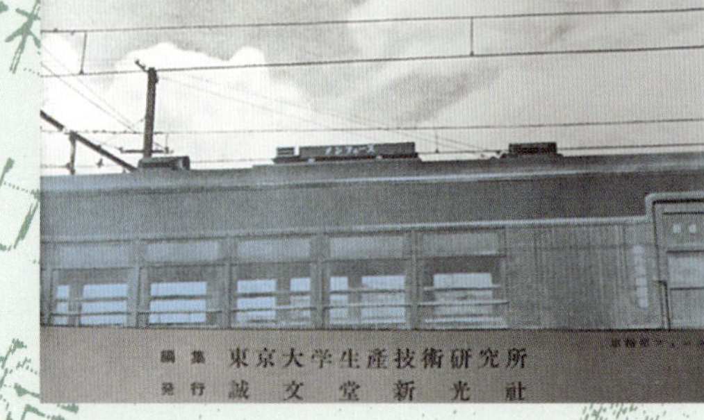
第2巻　第2号
生産研究
2
1950
編集　東京大学生産技術研究所
発行　誠文堂新光社

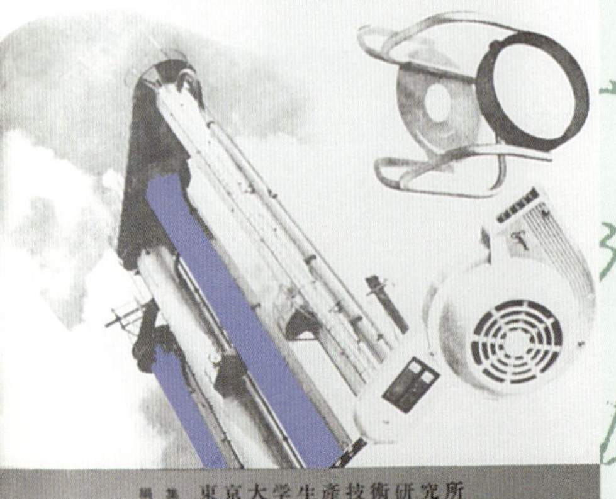
生産研究
第2巻　第11号
"合成樹脂の応用"
特集号
11
1950
編集　東京大学生産技術研究所
発行　誠文堂新光社

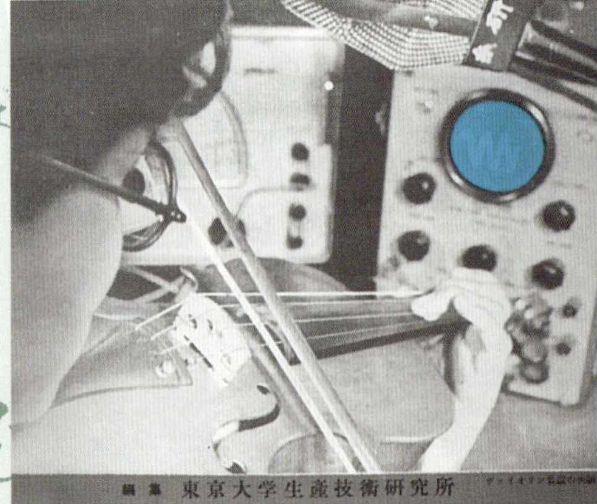
生産研究
3巻　第1号
1
1951
編集　東京大学生産技術研究所
発行　誠文堂新光社

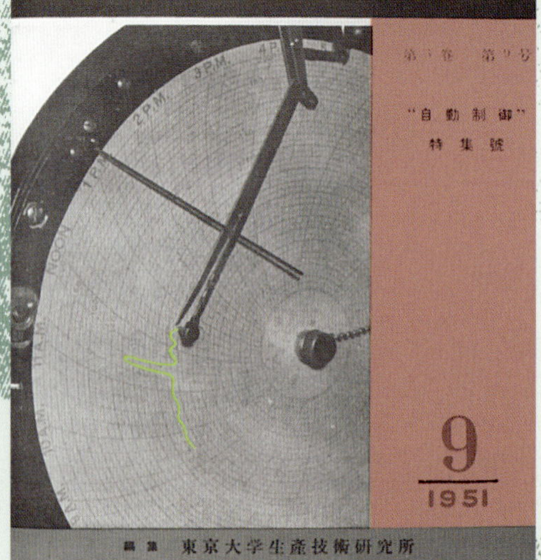
生産研究
第1巻　第9号
"自動制御"
特集號
9
1951
編集　東京大学生産技術研究所
発行　誠文堂新光社

I.I.S in Japan flourished with the postwar recovery period. The enthusiasm researchers felt in those days can be seen in the faces portrayed on the cover of the Institute's 'Seisan-Kenkyu' publication.

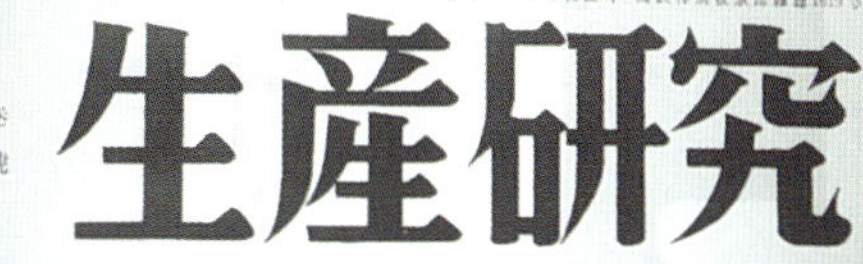

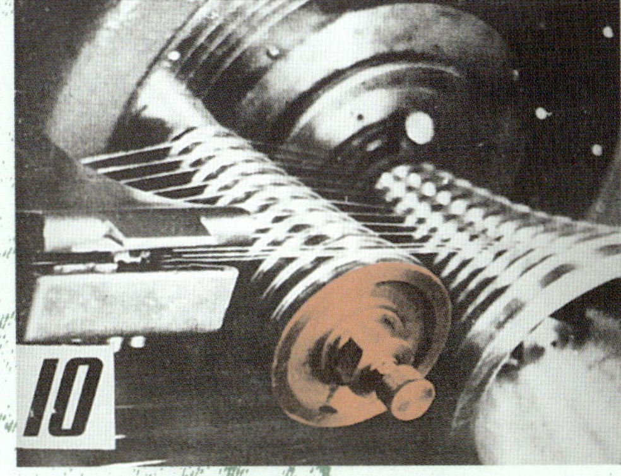

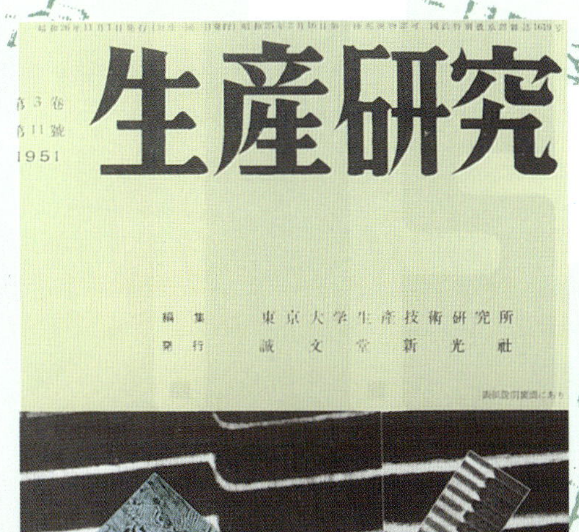

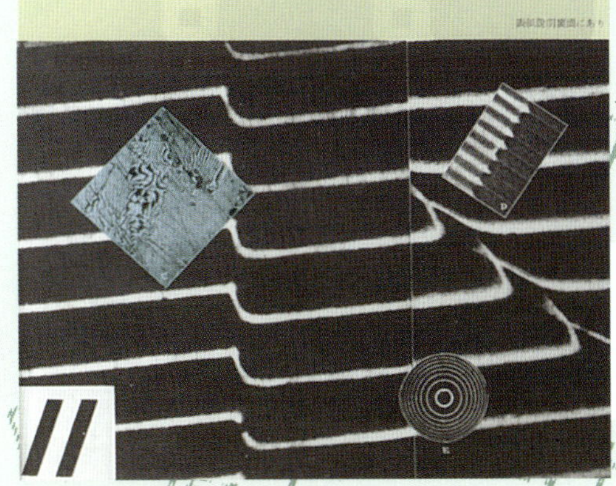

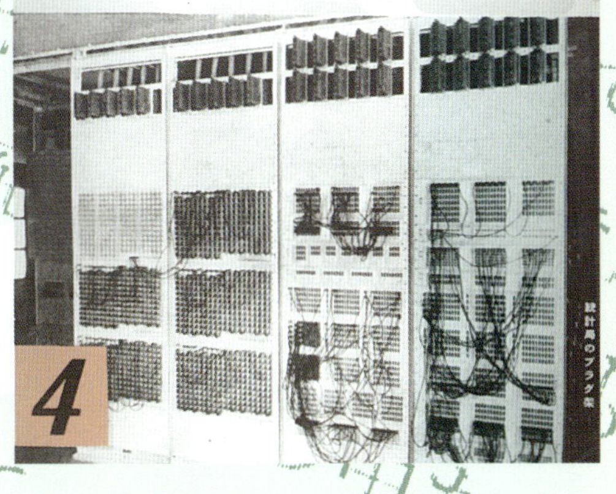

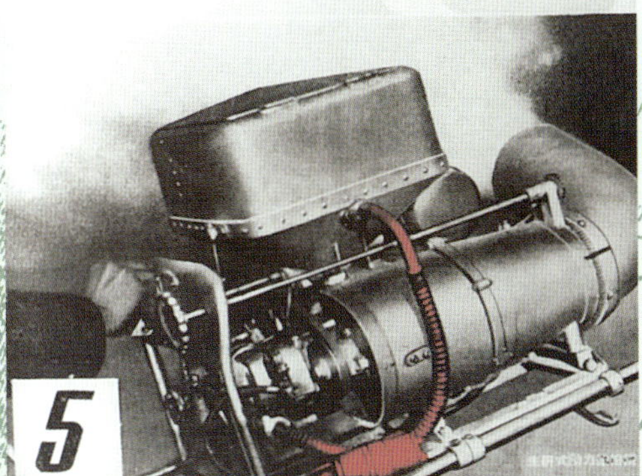

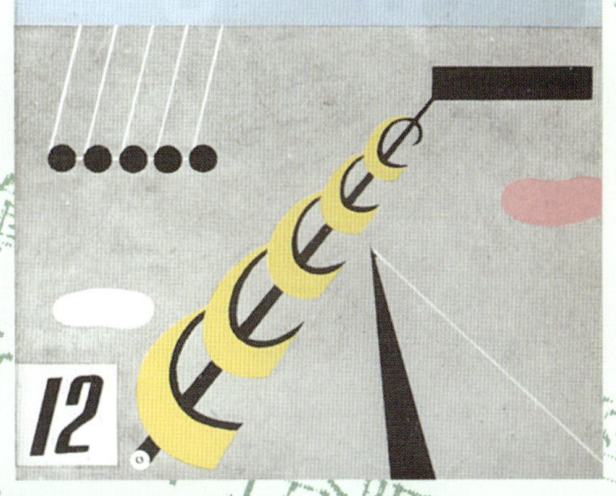

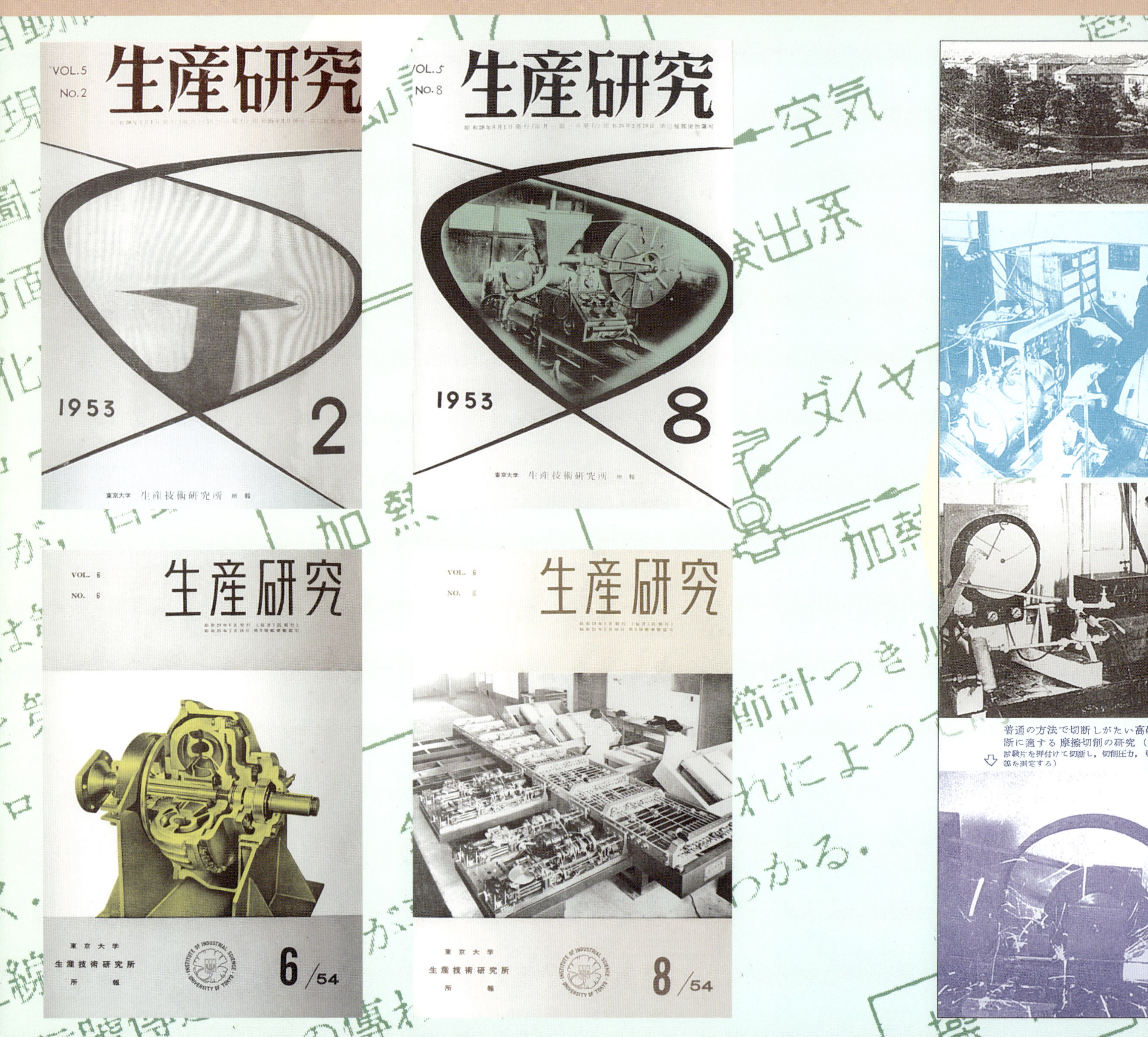

Research permeated Japanese society in the post-war era, leading to a new era of unparalleled economic growth. This period indirectly created the social environment into which the current generation of research leaders at I.I.S. was born.

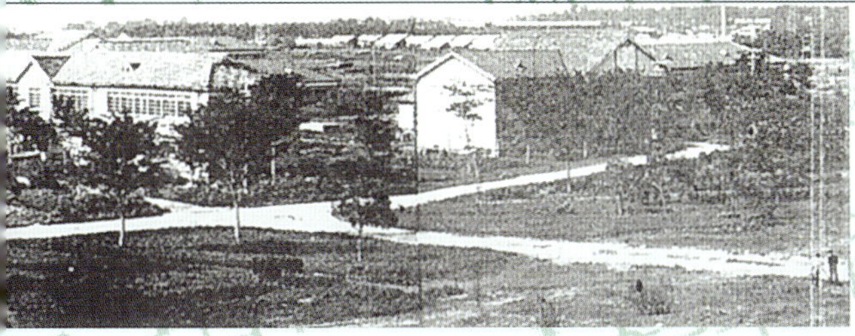

展望写眞：右方は第2部，中央前方は第1部，左方の建物はすべて第2部

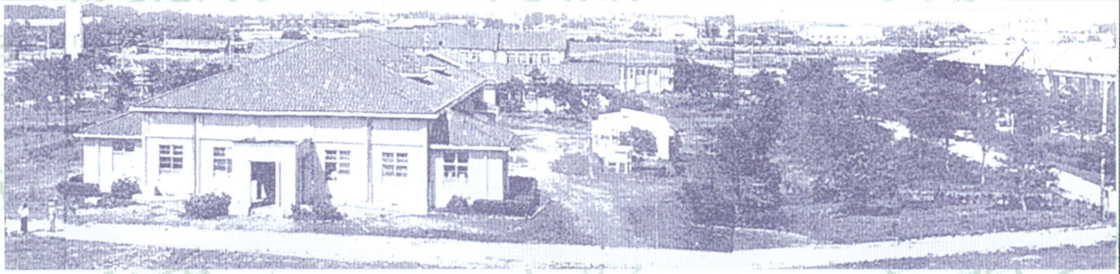

展望写真：前面の建物は講堂，そのうしろに食堂を隔てて中央講義室がある

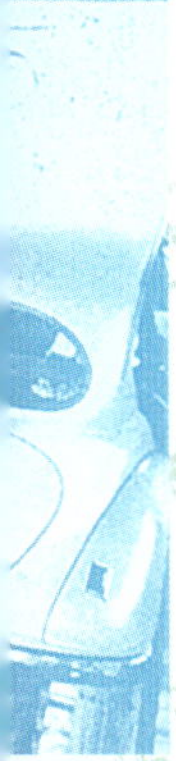

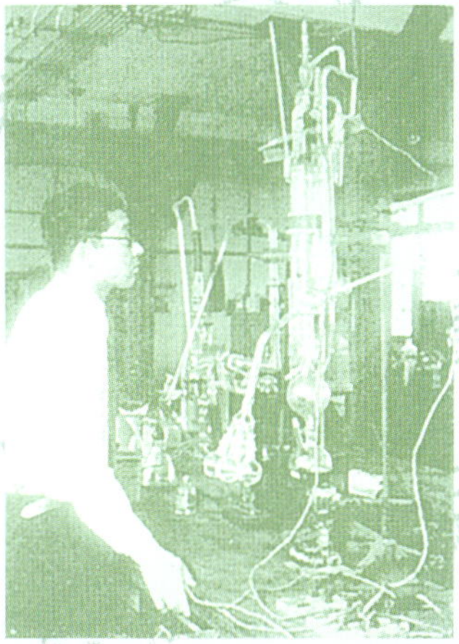

酸素製鉄試験設備
溶鉱炉底の溶鉄に酸素ガスを吹きこんで低珪，低硫黄の銑鉄をつくる

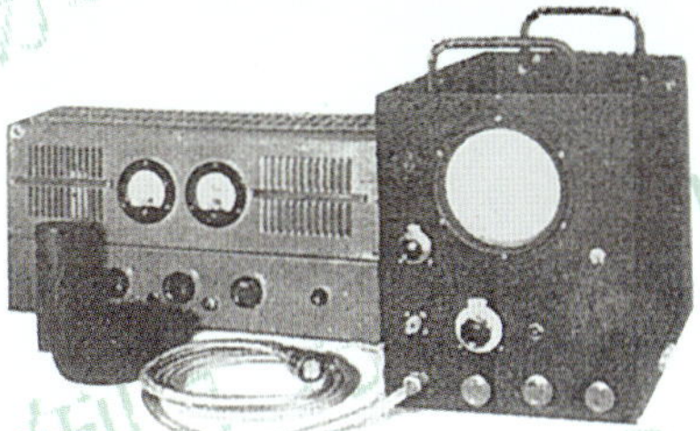

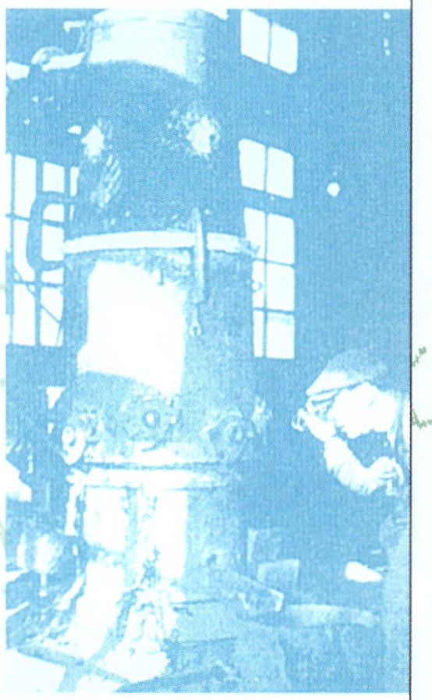

自動車試験台
直径約 1.4m の廻転ドラムに載せて各種の試験を行う　図は正弦カムを用いて馭装置の時性試験中の所

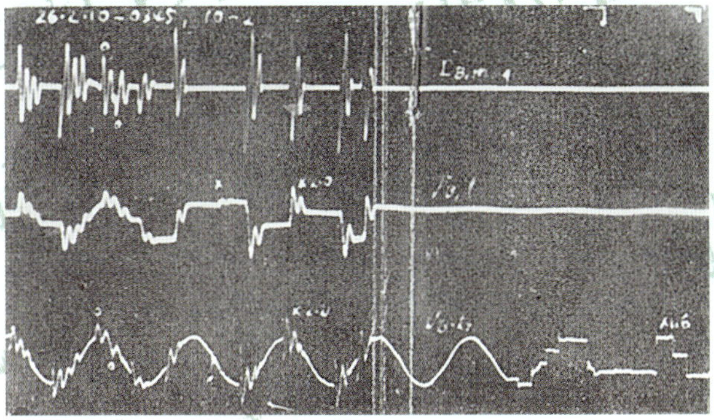

回転ドラム式3要素ブラウン管オシロクラン：
154,000 ボルト回路の遮断現象を撮影した一例
電圧波形に再点弧に伴う急峻な振動が見られる

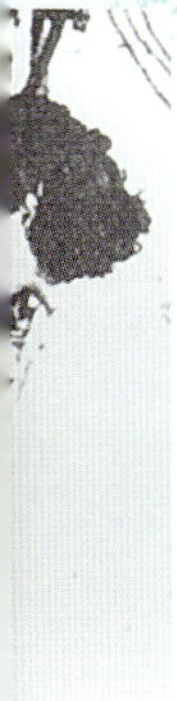

分子蒸溜装置
高度の眞空下で分子間相互の衝突を防ぎ凝集させて異種分子の分離を行うもので油脂・ヴィタミンの研究に多く用いる

正弦波挿入による自動調節計の試験：
周期 20秒〜20分のシグナル発振器によって自動調節計や工業プロセスの動特性を周波特性からしらべる

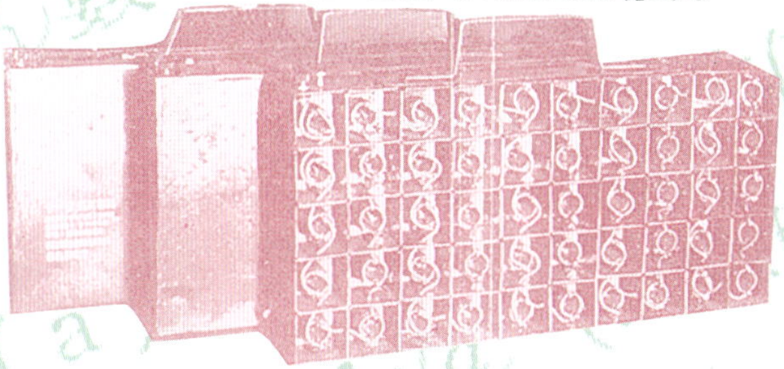

サージ遅延回路：
雷のような現象によって突然発生する電圧を記録しやすくするために，その波形を $5\mu s$ だけおくらせる装置

金属製品の中にある傷を外側から発見する超音波探傷器：検査したい材料の材質，傷の種類に応じ波長を連続的にかえることができる

液体ホーニング実験装置
（円壔状試験片に砥粒を含む噴流をあてて，表面を仕上げているところ）

4,000 MC 誘電体特性測定装置
波長 7.5cm（周波数 4,000 MC）の超高周波における電気絶縁物の誘電体特性 ε, $\tan\delta$ の測定装置で，高周波ケーブル，碍子の減衰測定，金属板表面損失の測定にも応用することができる

分光分析装置
左方が水晶分光写真器，右方がミクロフォトメーターで，金属などを分析する

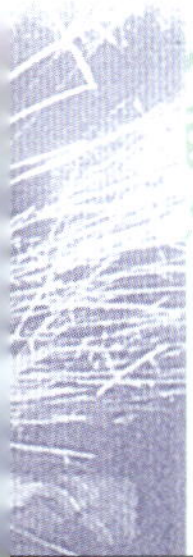

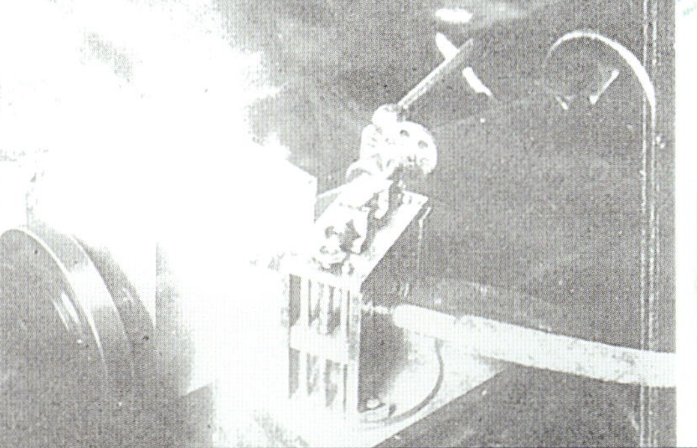

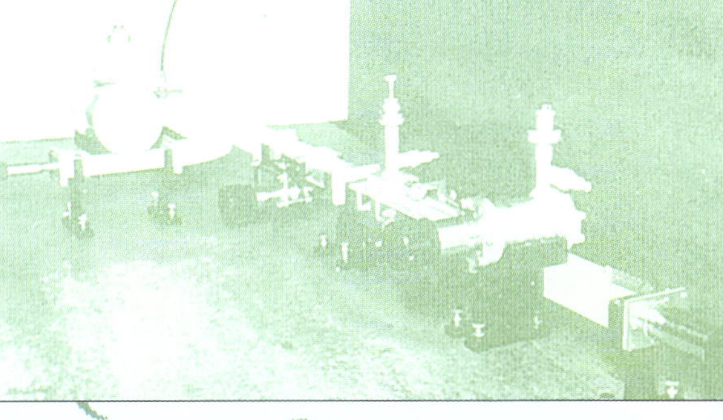

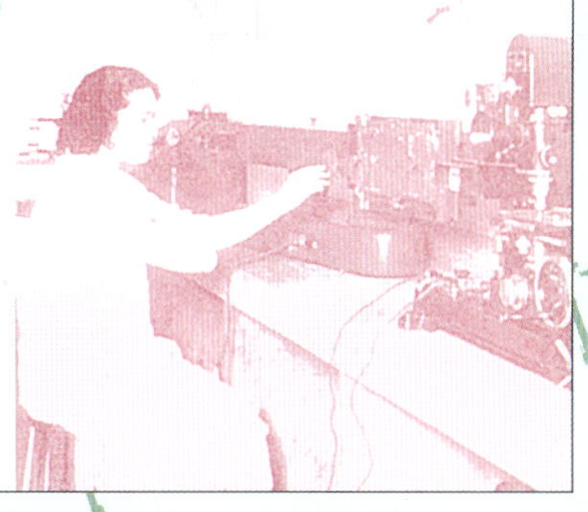

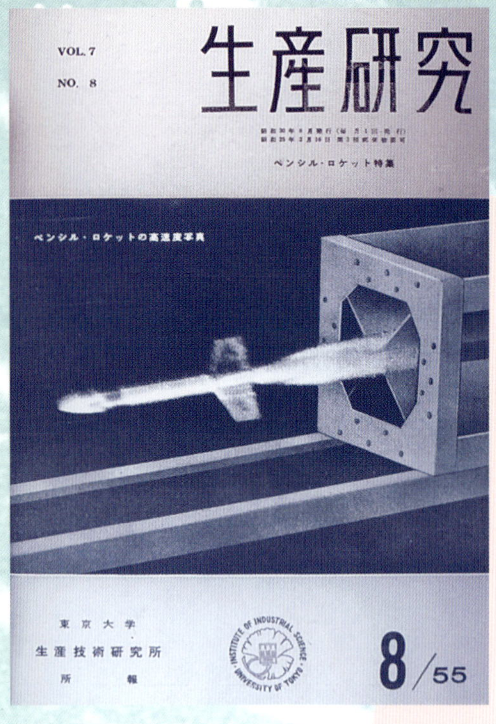

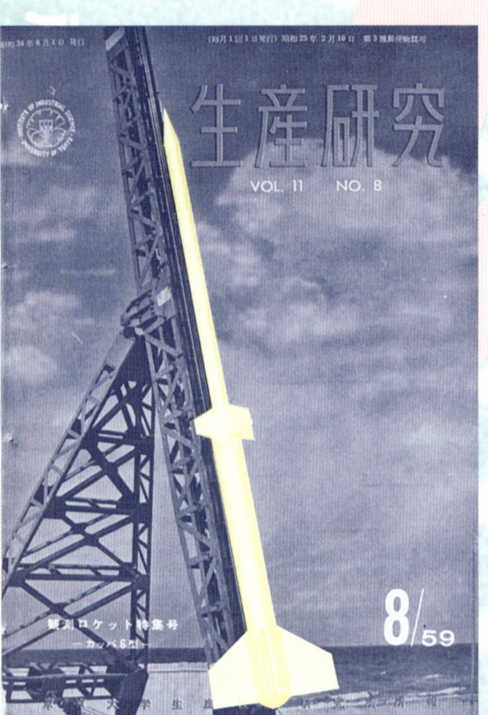

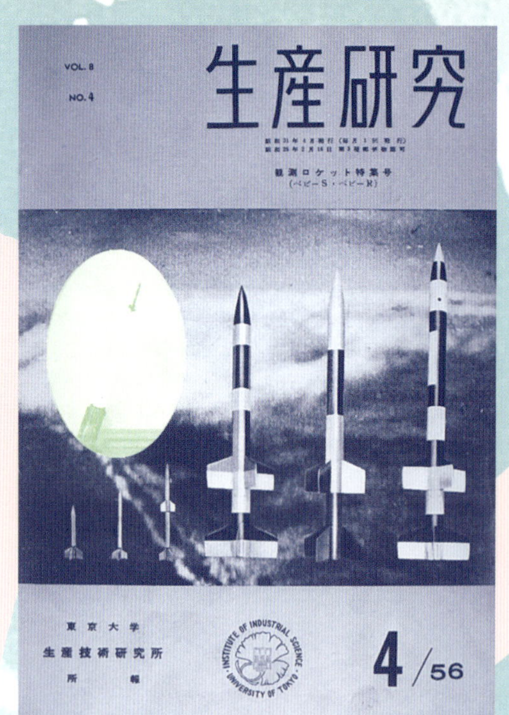

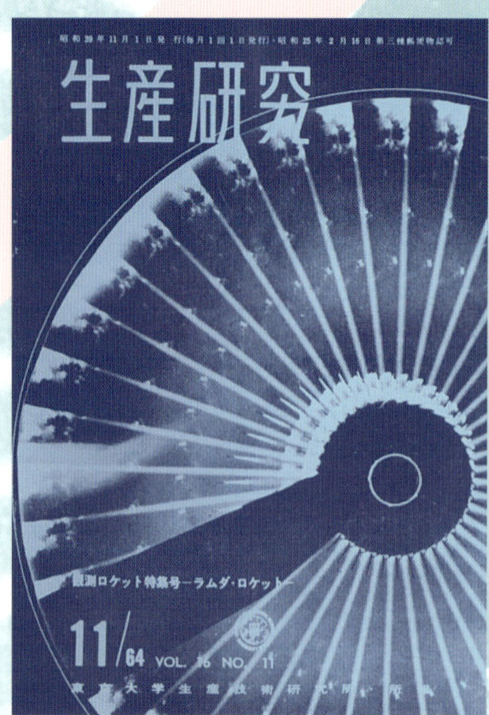

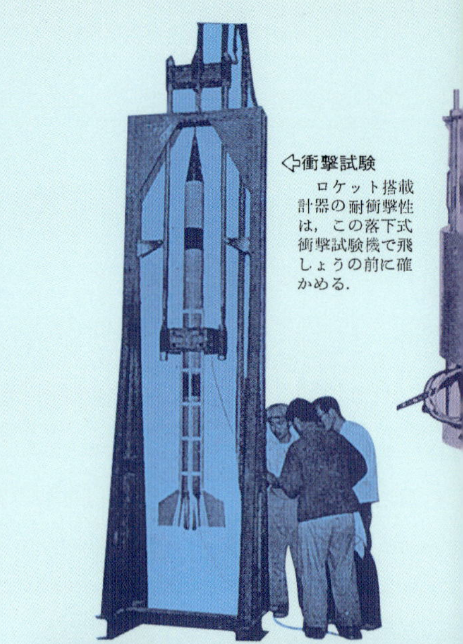

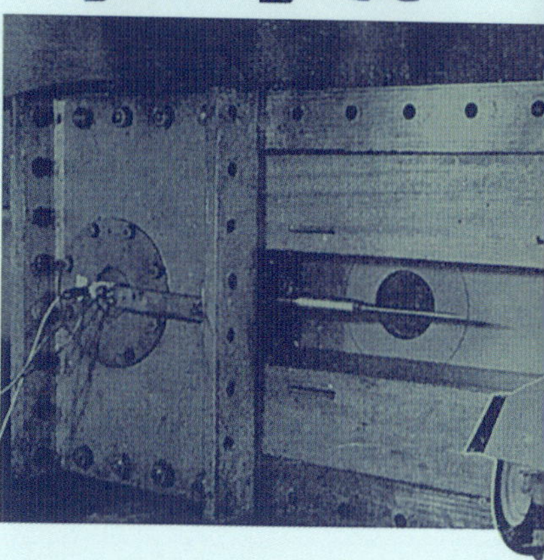

　1957〜58 年の 国際地球観測年 に使用する観測用ロケットの製作を東京大学生産技術研究所が行うことになり，昭和 30 年より研究に着手し，ペンシル，ベビー・ロケットにつづきカッパ・ロケットの試作および試験が行われております．

　糸川研究室では，ロケットの研究としてロケット用固体燃料および燃焼に関する基礎的研究,ロケットの性能,安定，力学に関する研究，およびロケットの設計法に関する理論的ならびに実験的研究が行われています．またロケットの飛しょう性能を測定するため，ロケットに搭載する加速度計，減速度計，および気圧高度計の研究試作も行っています．

　玉木研究室ではロケットの空気力学に関する研究を行

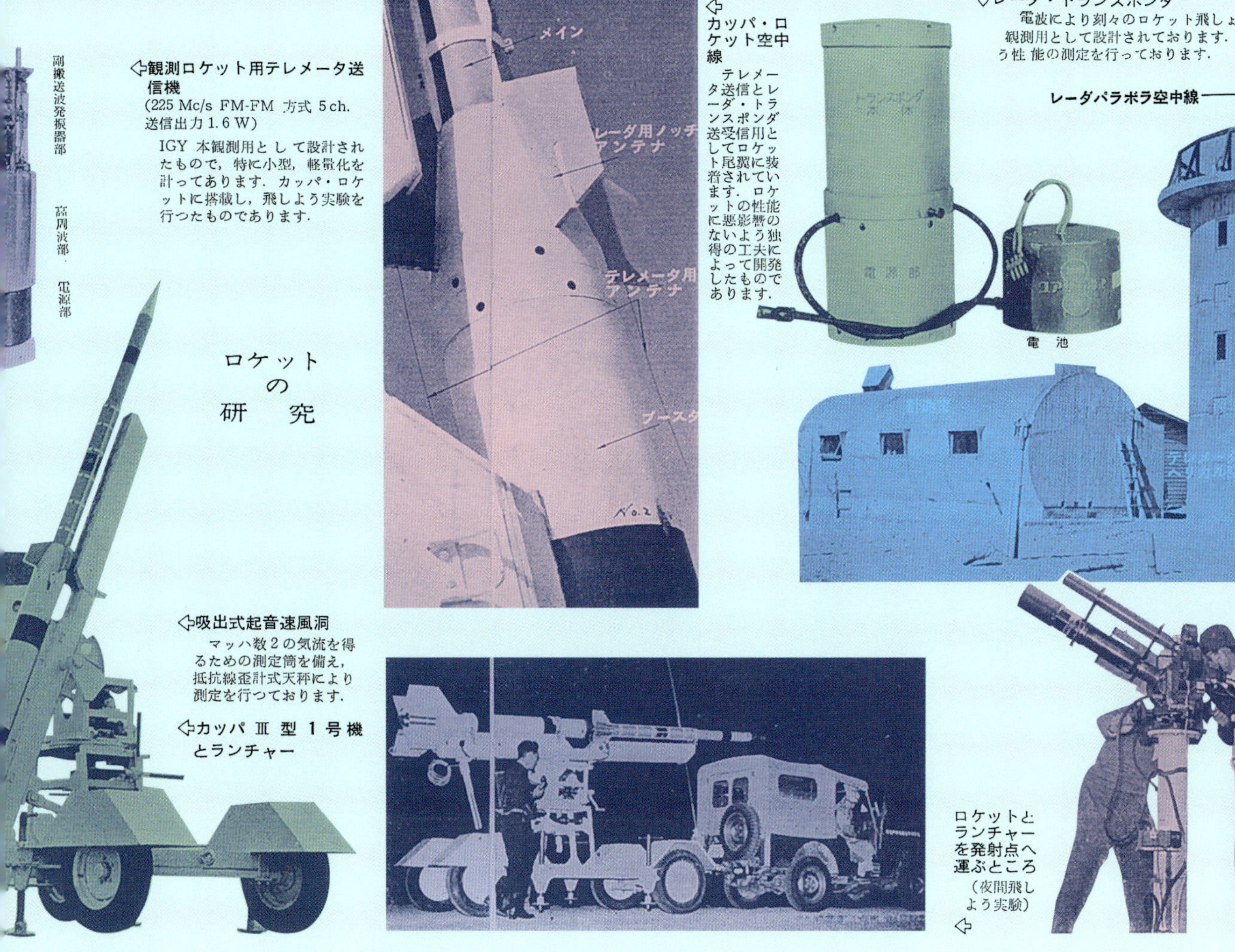

間欠送波発振器部

高周波部・電源部

◁観測ロケット用テレメータ送信機
（225 Mc/s FM-FM 方式 5 ch. 送信出力 1.6 W）
IGY本観測用として設計されたもので，特に小型，軽量化を計ってあります．カッパ・ロケットに搭載し，飛しよう実験を行つたものであります．

ロケットの研究

◁吸出式超音速風洞
マッハ数2の気流を得るための測定筒を備え，抵抗線歪計式天秤により測定を行つております．

◁カッパ III 型 1 号機とランチャー

◁カッパ・ロケット空中線
テレメータ送信とレーダ・トランスポンダ送信用としてロケット尾翼に装着されています．ロケットの性能に悪影響のないよう独得の工夫によって開発したものであります．

⇩レーダ・トランスポンダ
電波により刻々のロケット飛しょう径路を測定するためのもので IGY本観測用として設計されております．カッパ・ロケットに搭載し，その飛しよう性能の測定を行っております．

◁観測室と計測室の全景
テレメータ受信およびレーダ観測装置が設置してあります．屋上にレーダ用パラボラ空中線，建物の前面にテレメータ受信用ヘリカル空中線が置かれています．

ロケットの光学的観測
ロケットの飛しょう状況を観測・追跡撮影するためにロケット実験場周辺に数個所に各種光学的追跡装置が設けられています．⇩

ロケットとランチャーを発射点へ運ぶところ
（夜間飛しよう実験）◁

低速および高速風洞における風洞試験，安定計算，計算などを行っています．

…田研究室では，翼の静的強さとフラッタ・燃焼室・部およびノーズコーンの強さなどについて主として的研究を行い，またランチャーの構造法の研究法もました．森研究室も池田研究室と協力し特にロケット振動関係を担当しております．

…村研究室では，ロケットなどの高速飛しよう体の光追跡用装置，ならびに応用に関する研究を行つてお当研究所観測ロケット班の一員として，高速度撮影追跡用シネオドライト装置ロケット搭載用特殊などの製作研究を行い，これらを使用してロケット飛しよう特性の解析を行つております．

また丸安研究室でも，橱村研究室と協力してロケットの光学的追跡の研究を行つております．

高木・野村・黒川研究室では，観測ロケット用エレクトロニクス装置の研究を行つております．テレメータ装置では，本観測用受信記録装置が完成し，現在，秋田（道川）実験場に設置されております．またテレメータ送信機も初期のものに比べると，極めて小型軽量化に成功しました．その性能をさらに向上するためにトランジスタ化の研究も進めております．

また，ロケットの飛しよう径路測定のために，自動追跡レーダを初め，種々の電波標定装置が開発されました．ロケットに搭載するレーダ・トランスポンダも軽量小型のものが完成しております．

ロケット用空中線は，ロケット搭載機器の性能を大きく支配しますが，これについても新しい独自の方式のものが開発されています．これらの各種エレクトロニクス装置は数次にわたるカッパ・ロケットの飛しよう実験において，いずれも優秀な性能を発揮することを確めております．

富永研究室では，ロケットに乗せる気圧計の研究，試作を行つています．

またこれらの研究室のほかに，ロケット飛しよう実験のときの地上測量を丸安研究室が，秋田（道川）実験場の各種建築物（テストスタンド・計測室・準備室・レーダ室）などの設計を坪井・池辺研究室が，また実験時の通信連絡を第3部各研究室が担当しております．

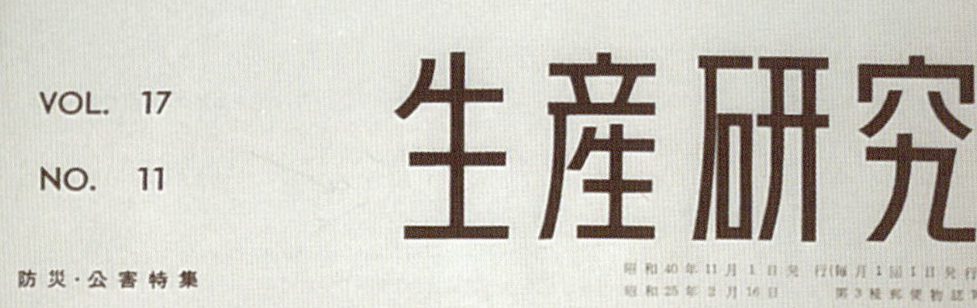
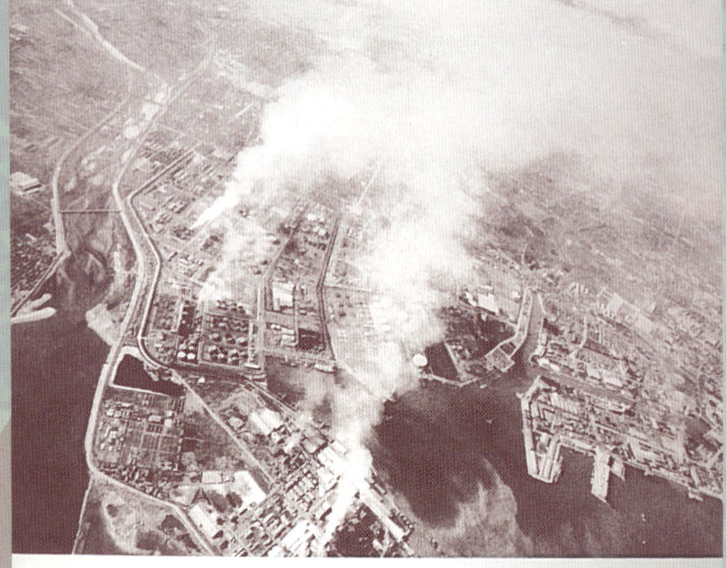
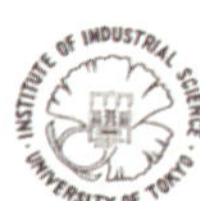
VOL. 17
NO. 11
生産研究
防災・公害特集
東京大学
生産技術研究所
所報
INSTITUTE OF INDUSTRIAL SCIENCE
UNIVERSITY OF TOKYO
11/65

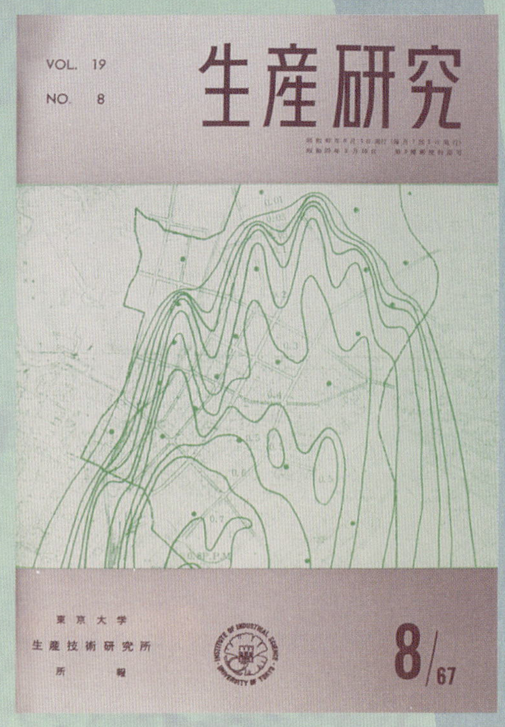
VOL. 19
NO. 8
生産研究
東京大学
生産技術研究所
所報
INSTITUTE OF INDUSTRIAL SCIENCE
UNIVERSITY OF TOKYO
8/67

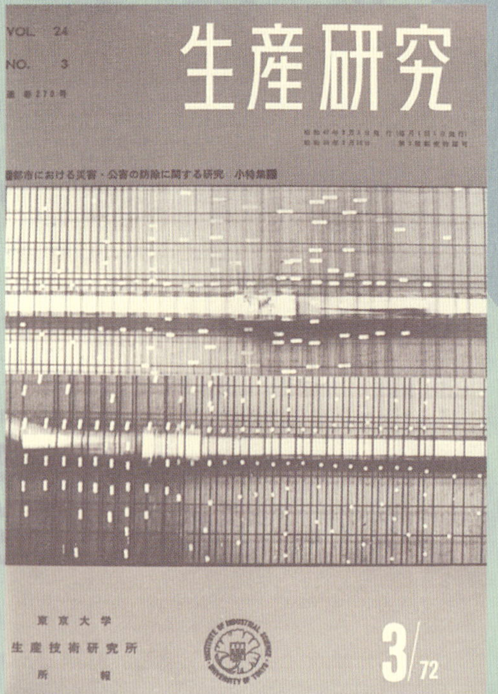
VOL. 24
NO. 3
生産研究
東京大学
生産技術研究所
所報
INSTITUTE OF INDUSTRIAL SCIENCE
UNIVERSITY OF TOKYO
3/72

As Japan experienced rapid economic growth, the issue of pollution surfaced as a major problem. A new, pollution-free paradigm and other new paradigms are needed for the future, since pollution is in no way an issue of the past.

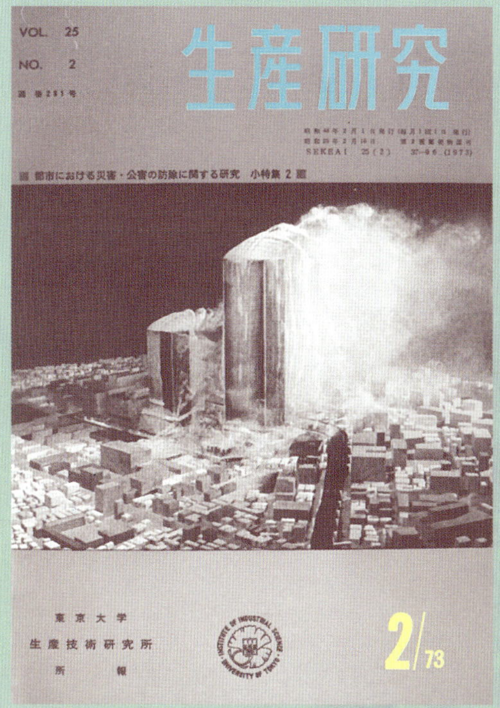

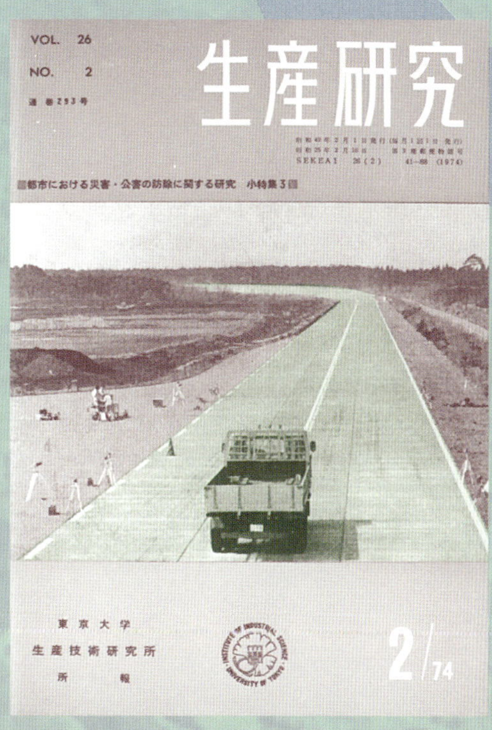

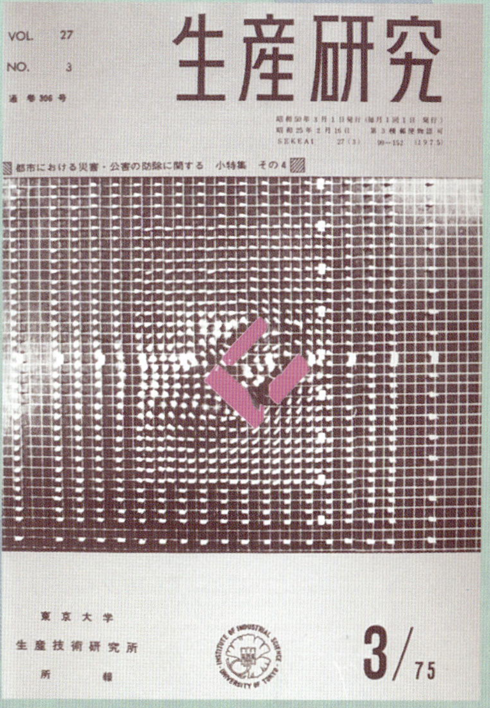

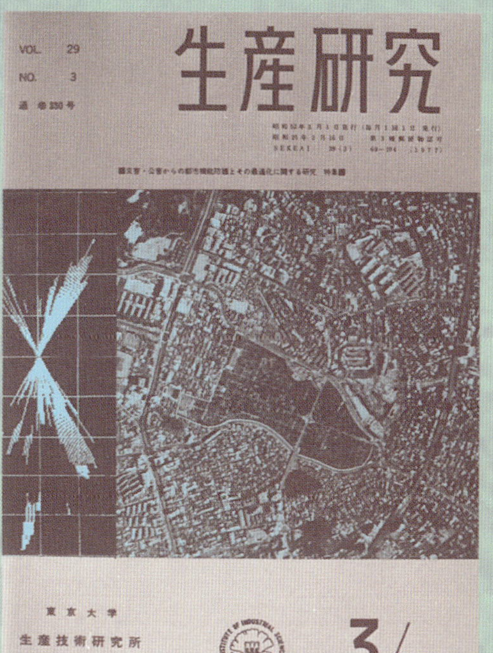

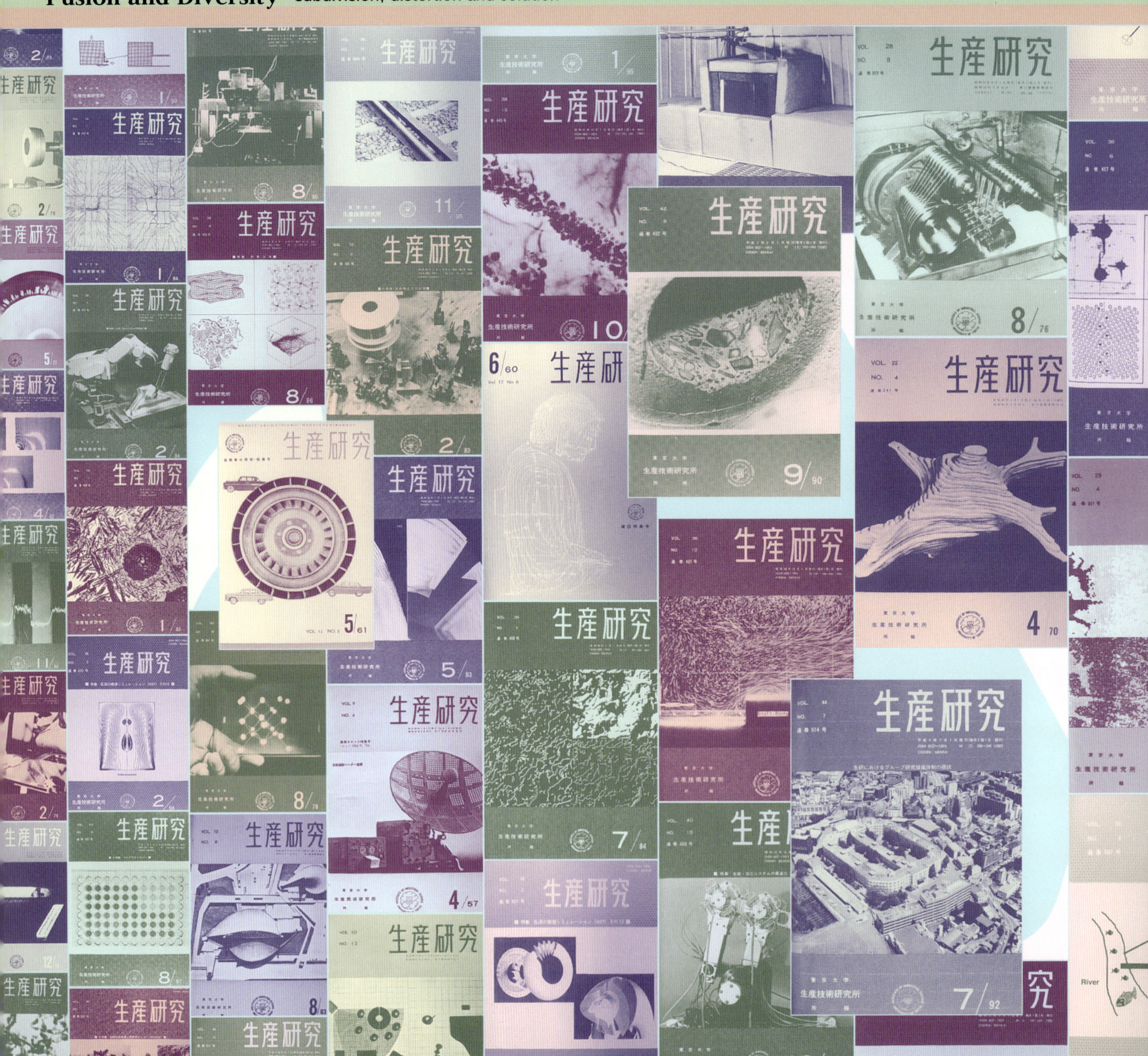

The new paradigms will appear in relation to those of the past. Research will inevitably become more diversified as the old and new converge. Whether we can cope with this added diversity is a critical question in modern engineering.

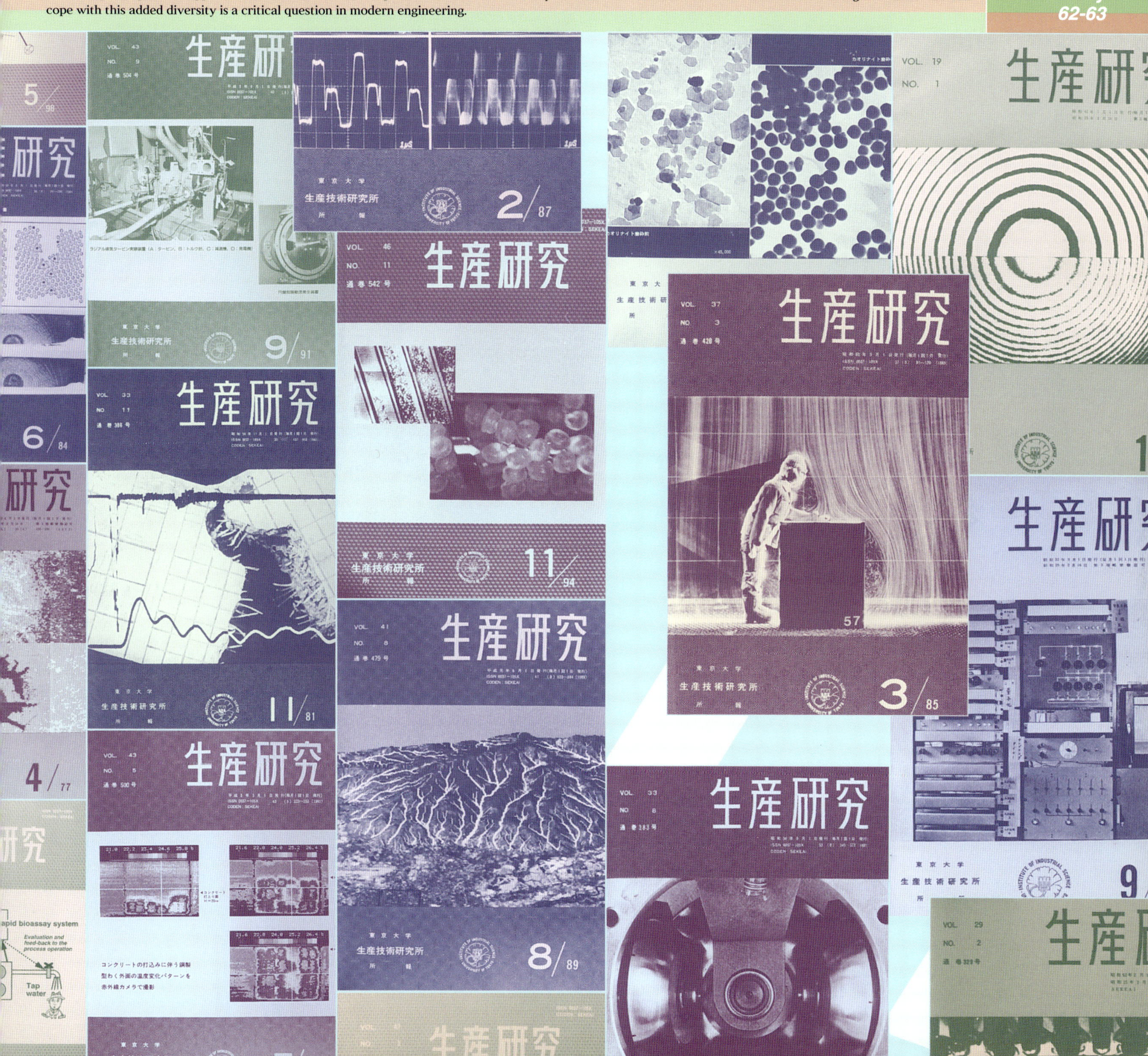

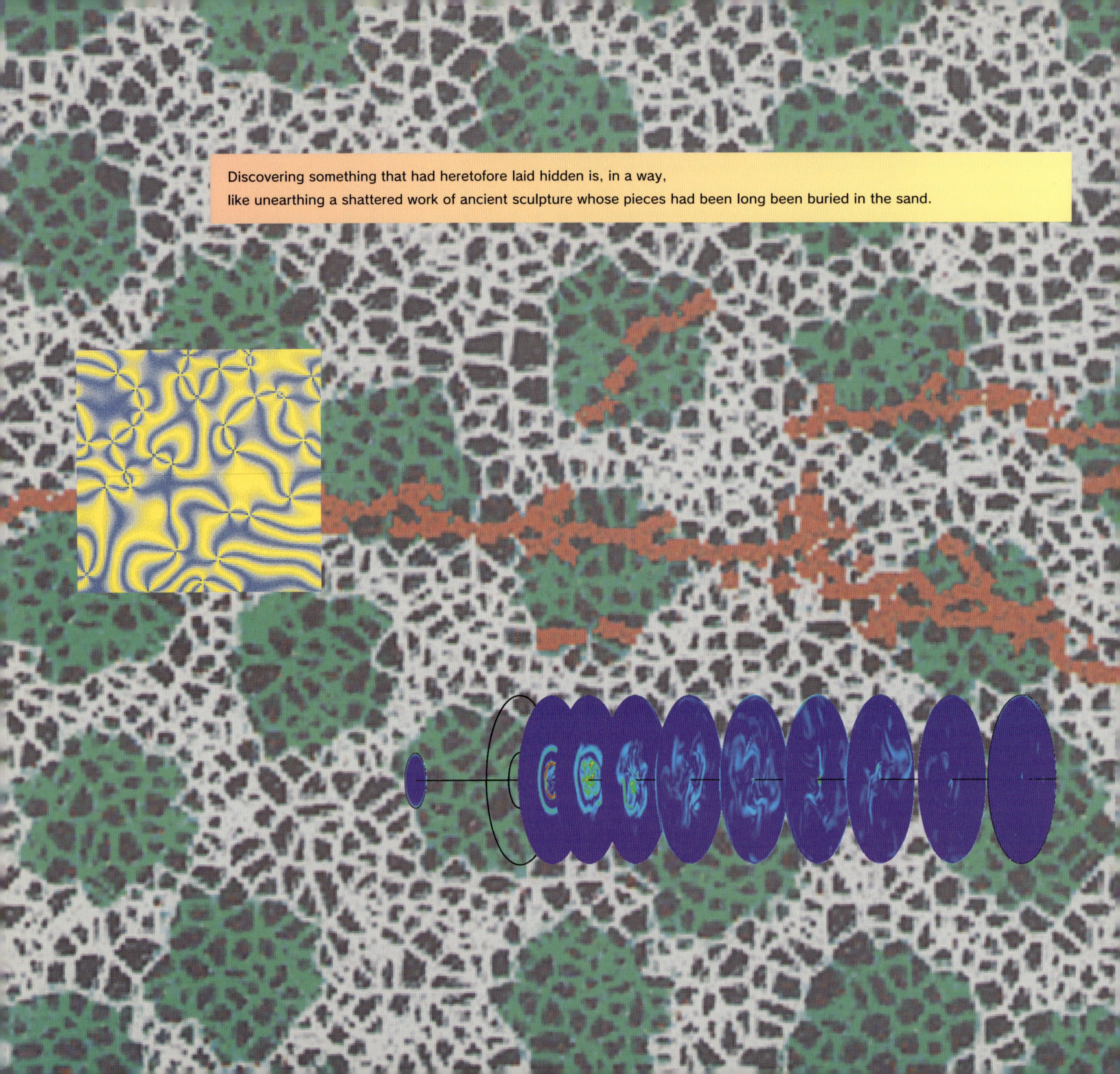

Discovering something that had heretofore laid hidden is, in a way,
like unearthing a shattered work of ancient sculpture whose pieces had been long been buried in the sand.

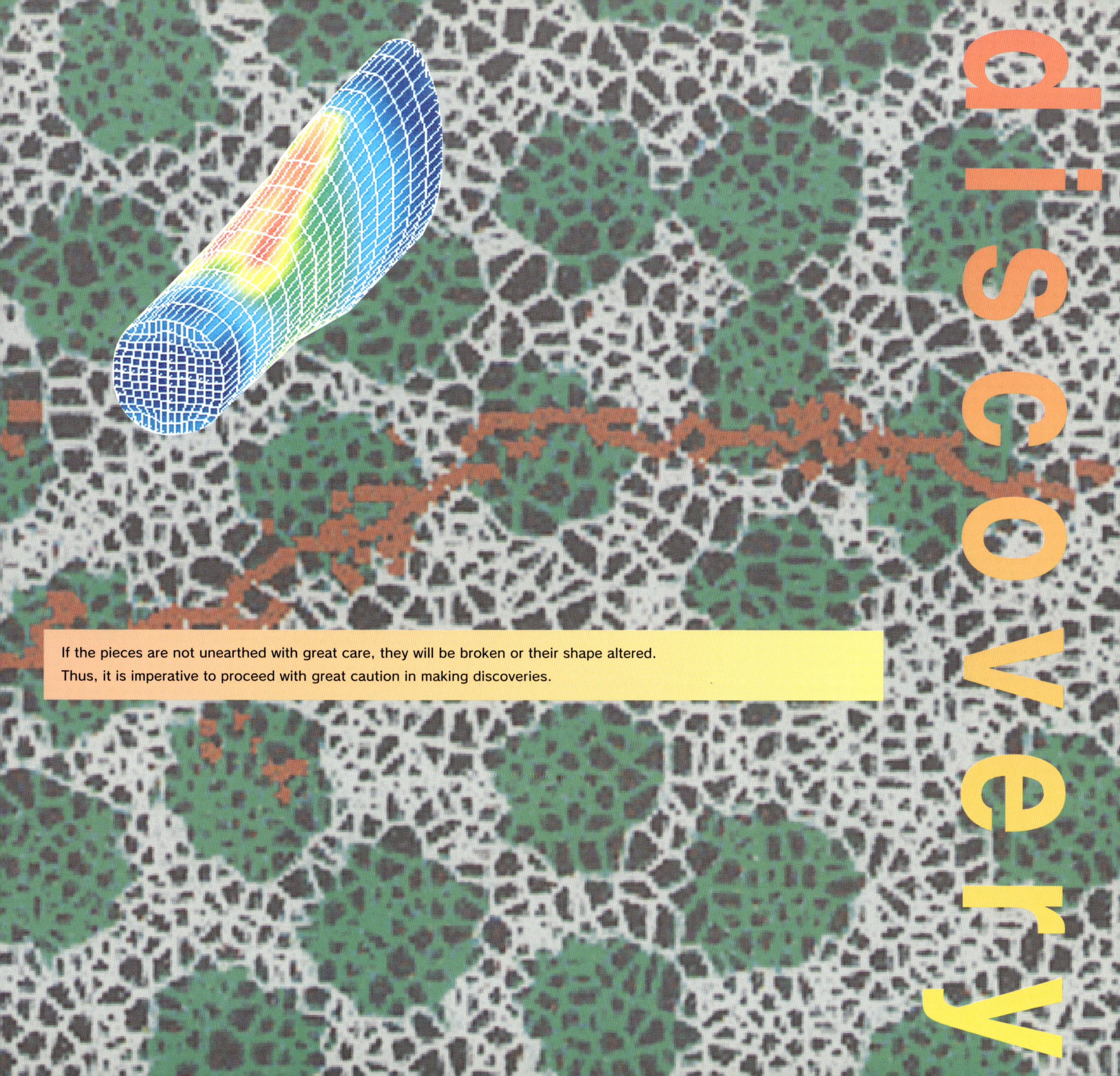

discovery
If the pieces are not unearthed with great care, they will be broken or their shape altered.
Thus, it is imperative to proceed with great caution in making discoveries.

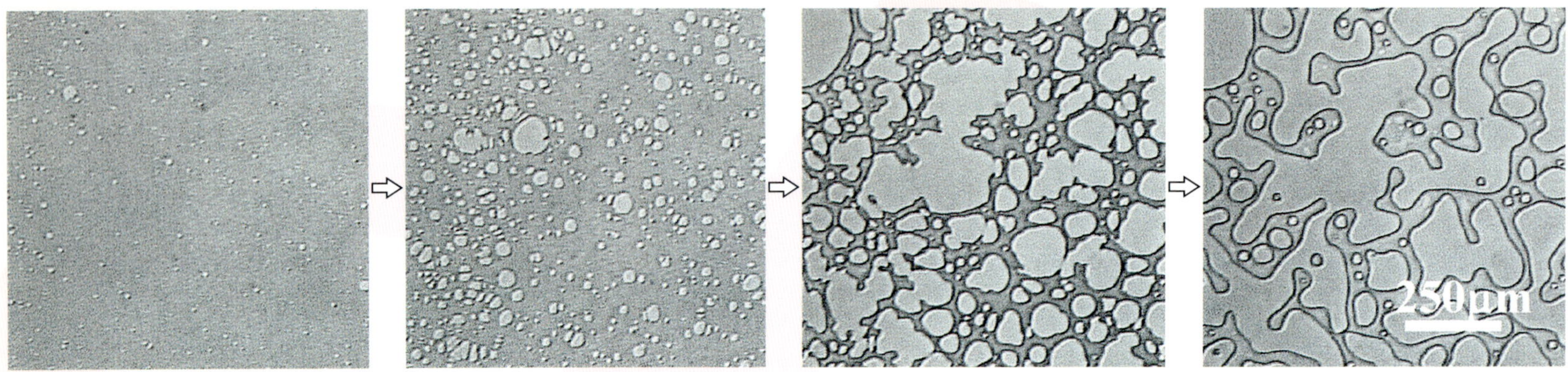

A new phase-separation model of condensed matter — Viscoelastic phase separation

Phase separation takes place in some binary mixtures such as a mixture of water and oil. Unusual phase separation is found in polymer solutions, which is composed of large chain-like (slow) molecules and small liquid (fast) molecules. Contrary to common belief, a minority phase appears as a network-like structure instead of as droplets. This is a new kind of phase separation of condensed matter.

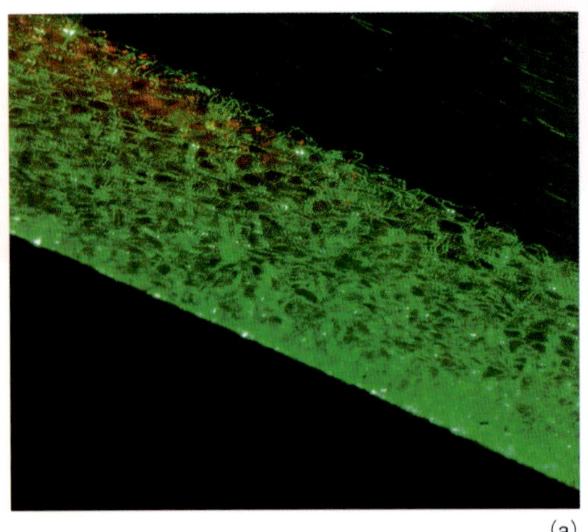

(a)

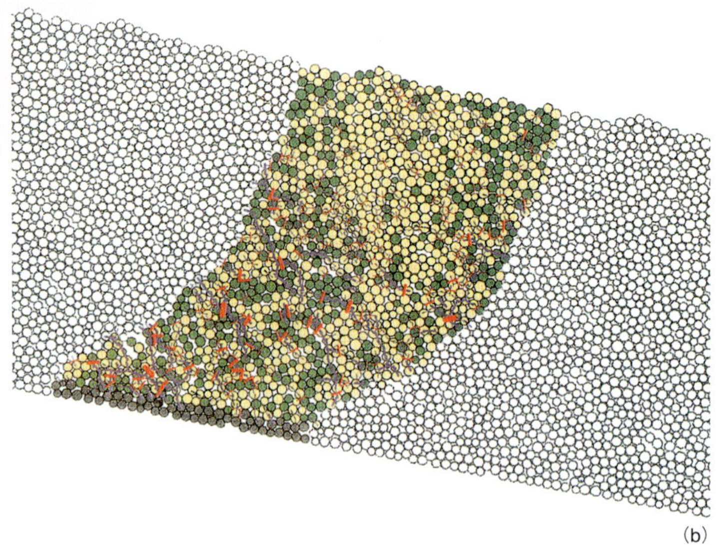

(b)

Shear-banding process in the interior of a granular slope model and its numerical simulation

Two powerful tools for studying grain-to-grain interaction in a granular assemblage have been developed; Laser-Aided Tomography (LAT, fig. (a)), allowing a cross-section of a granular slope to be visualized, and the Discrete Element Method (DEM, fig. (b)) for numerical simulations. Both methods enable us to follow all grains' motions in the interiors of granular assemblages, and thus provide important information on changes in granular fabrics.

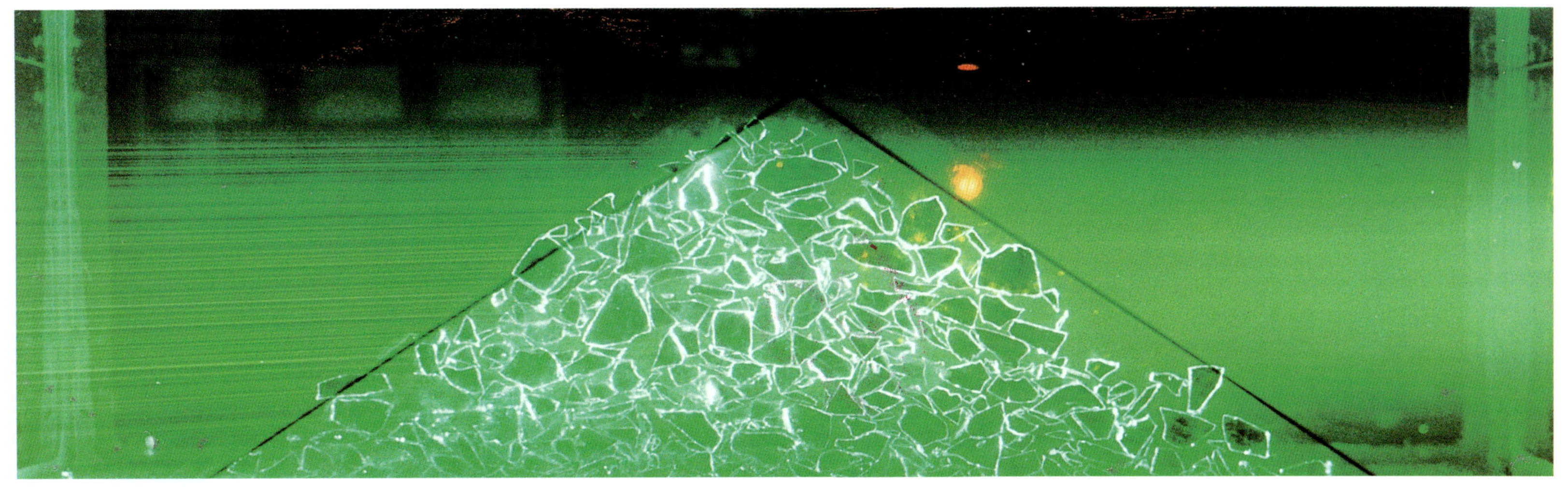

Cross section of a granular structure model visualized by LAT

You can look up at twinkling stars which are billions of light-year distances or farther, but you realize you cannot see any grains one inch deep in soil. In Laser-Aided Tomography (LAT), a granular structure model made up of particles of crushed optical glass immersed in a liquid with the same refractive index becomes invisible. An intense Laser-Light Sheet (LLS) is then passed through the model illuminating the contours of all the particles on a cross section optically cut by the LLS. Thus, scanning the model with LLS enables us to observe a detailed picture of its deformation.

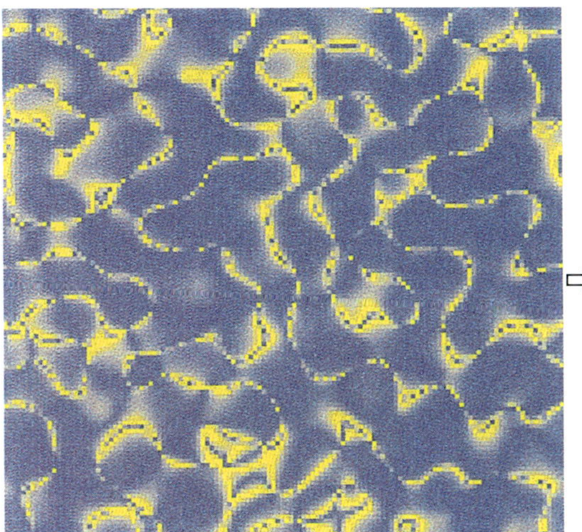 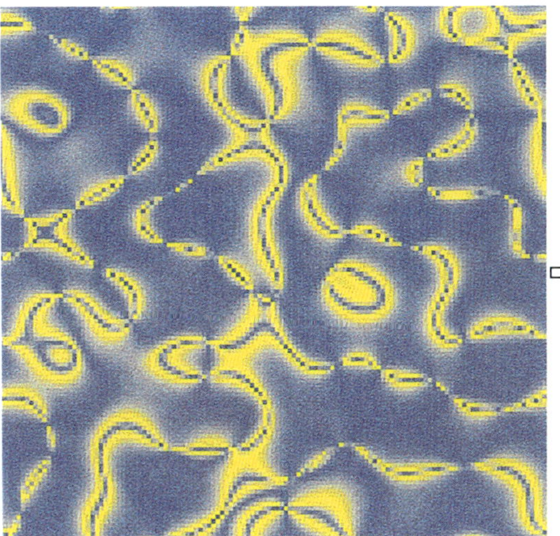 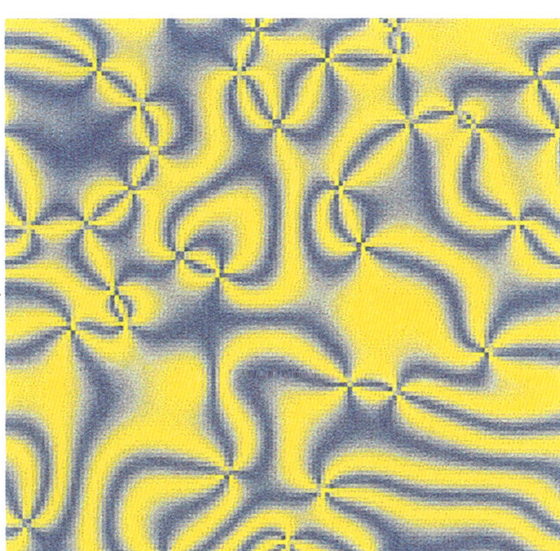

Isotropic-nematic phase transition of liquid crystal

A liquid crystalline phase such as a nematic phase is an intermediate phase existing between a liquid and crystal phase in some types of rod-like molecules. Numerical simulation of the isotropic-to-nematic transition process is performed. Just after the transition, many topological defects are created and then they gradually disappear to increase the orientational order.

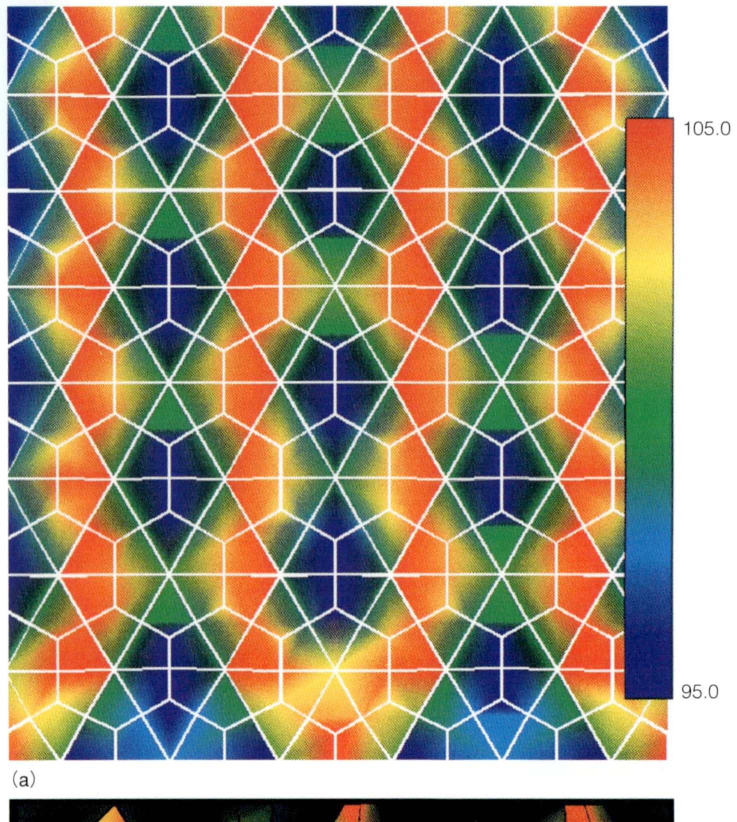

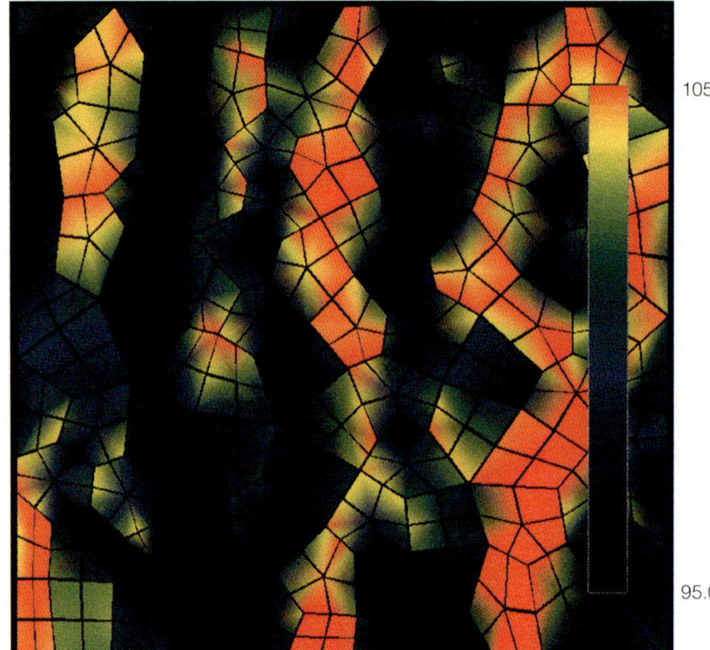

Stress analysis of polycrystalline solid

Ordinary materials are heterogeneous ones called polycrystalline, consisting of several 10 μm crystal grains. This heterogeneity is strongly related to the macroscopic strength of the materials. The pictures show the stress distributions in polycrystalline material at elevated temperatures evaluated by a unique numerical calculation technique. A higher irregularity of stress distribution can be observed in the model that has an irregular crystal grain (fig. (b)) compared with a regular hexagonal one (fig. (a)).

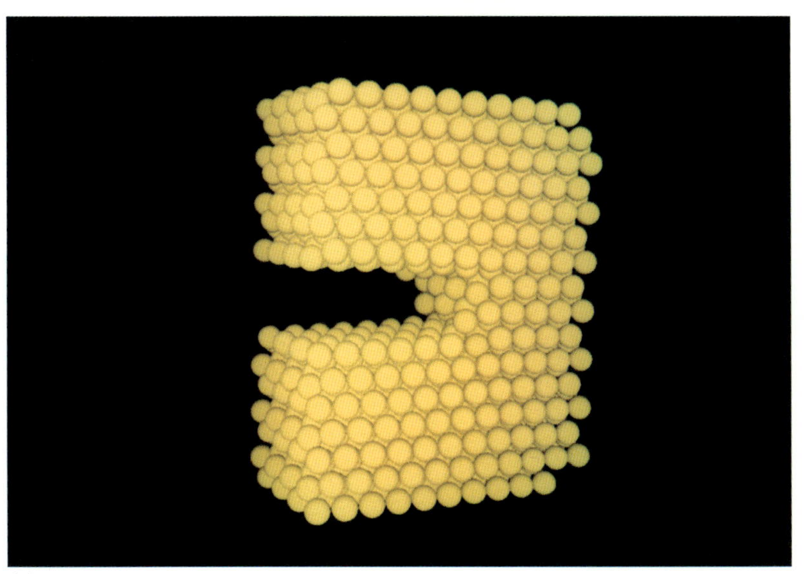

(a)

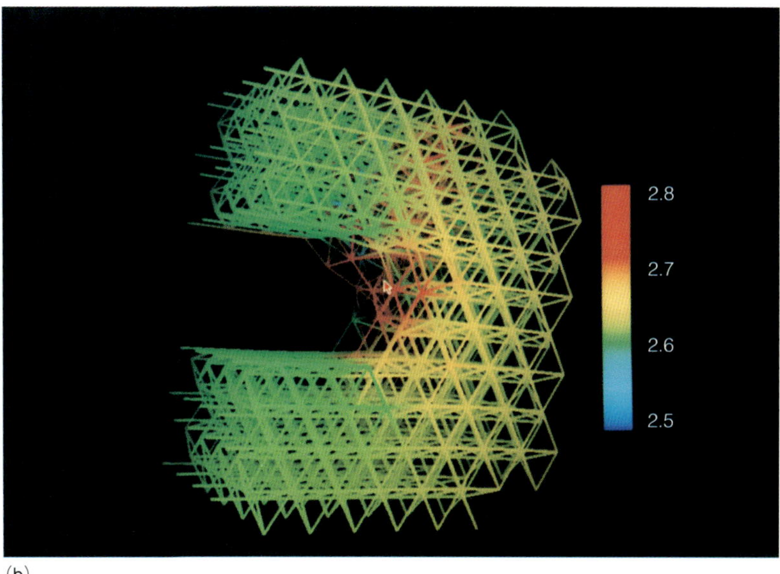

(b)

Crack analysis using an atomic array model

Of course all materials are an aggregate of microscopic atoms. When we want to discern the essentials of material failure, we finally arrive at the microscopic world. The pictures show the result of a simulation of atomic-scale crack behavior using the Molecular Dynamic Method. The atomic array configuration is shown in fig. (a), and the color variation in fig. (b) shows the magnitude of the force acting between the atoms.

Fracture simulation of fiber reinforced composite material

Advanced materials, which are reinforced with a kind of fiber are commonly used. As the failure processes of such materials are complicated, the evaluation of strength for such material is not so easy. The picture shows the result of crack growth simulation for ceramic fiber-reinforced material, and it is shown that the crack extension process is attended by pulled-out fiber bridging across the cracked plane.

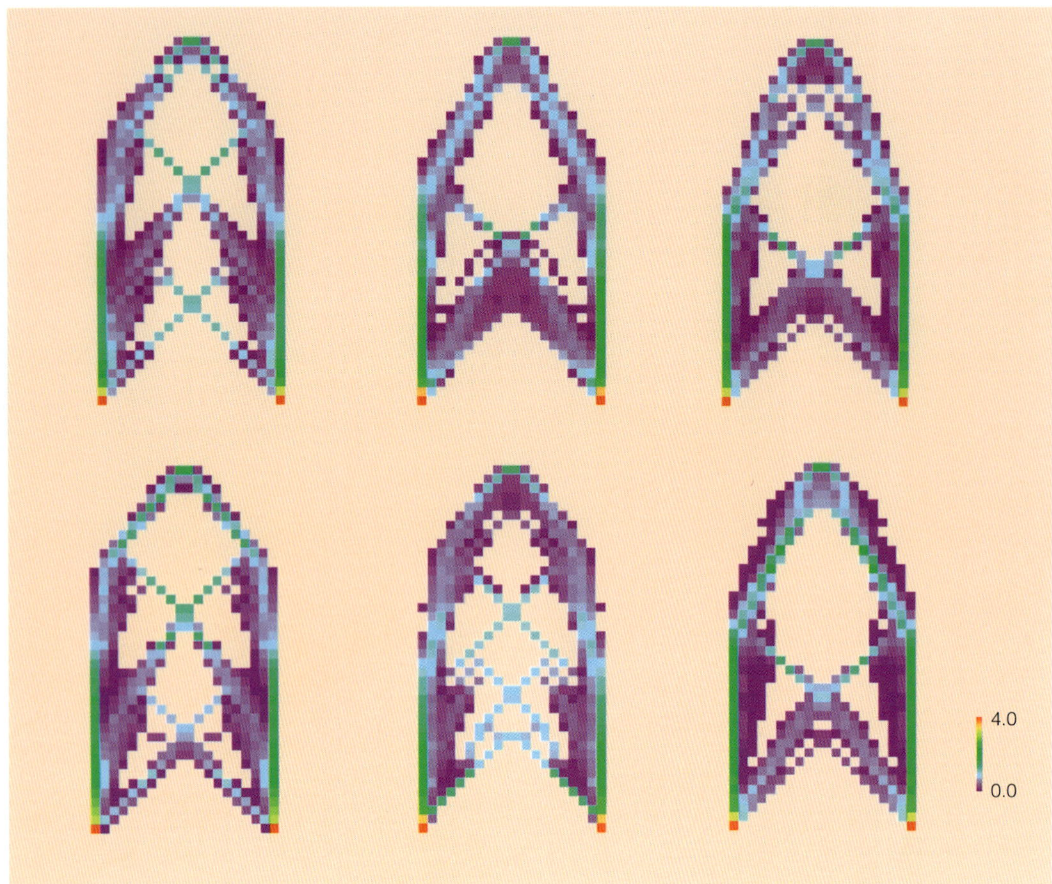

Optimum structural design by cellular automata

There has been a belief that a candidate for optimum structural design is obtained by the imitation of biological growth rules against external forces. Such rules can be described by cellular automata. A slight change of parameter value in the cellular automata gives rise to various shapes and topologies of structure, as is seen in the natural world.

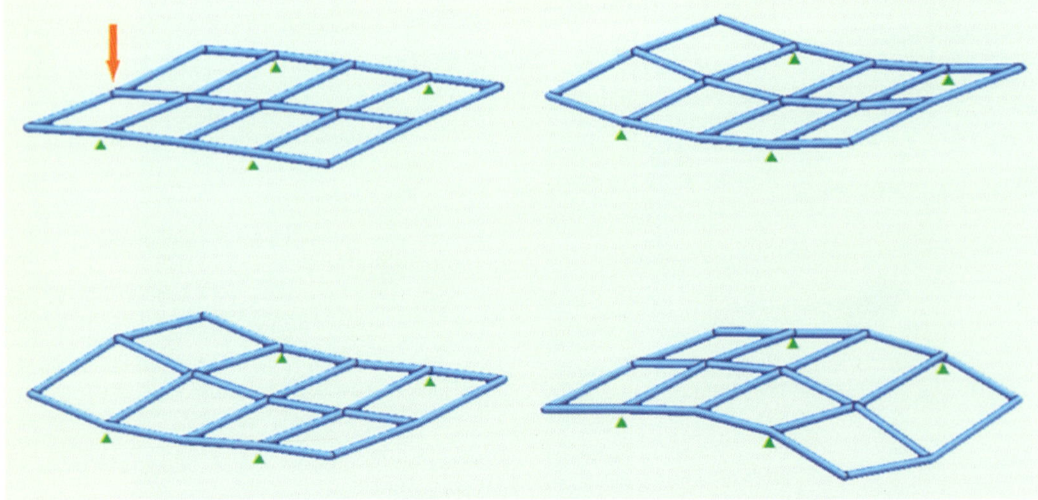

Homology design to virtually enhance structural stiffness

The geometrical property of a structure is kept before, during and after the deformation by homology design. A part of a structure can be virtually stiffened by means of this methodology, even where the structure becomes flexible caused by a light weight requirement. The center rib of a frame structure can be kept straight and virtually stiff under an excitation by this methodology.

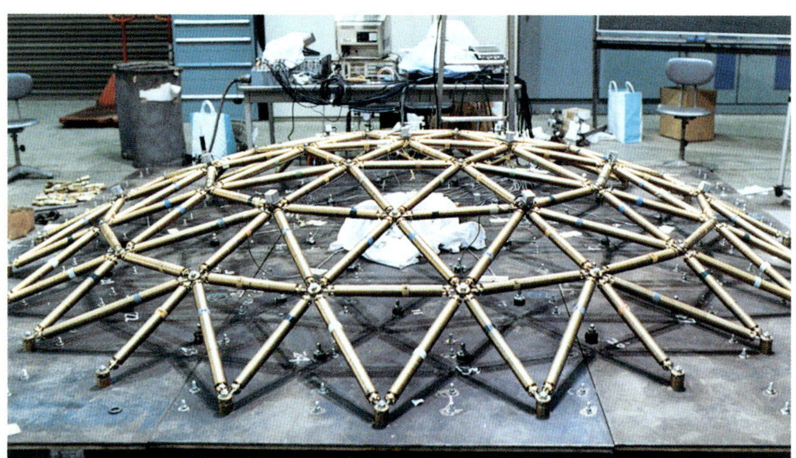

(a)

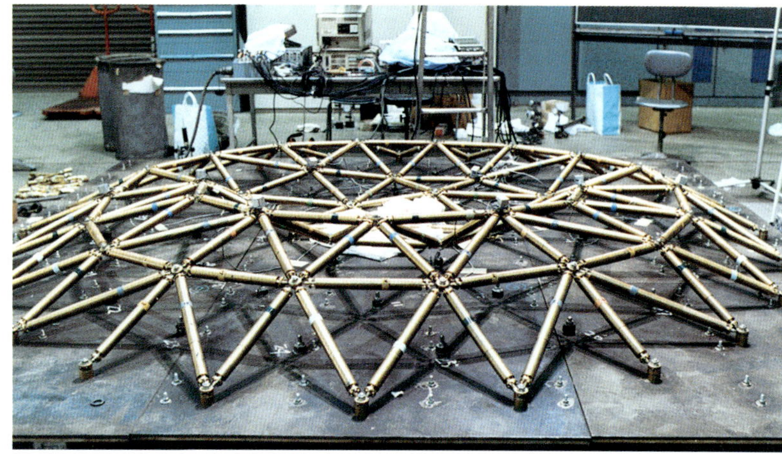

(b)

Vibration test of space frame on the shaking table

Because of its poor bending rigidity, a space frame should be carefully designed especially against buckling phenomena. The photos show the vibration test by vertical excitation on the shaking table, for the purpose of investigating the dynamic buckling of a single layer space frame under seismic ground motion. The natural frequencies are excited before the occurrence of dynamic buckling and the periodic vibration behavior is observed. However, near the dynamic buckling point, complicated coupled vibration arises because of its nonlinear effect, and it eventually fails.

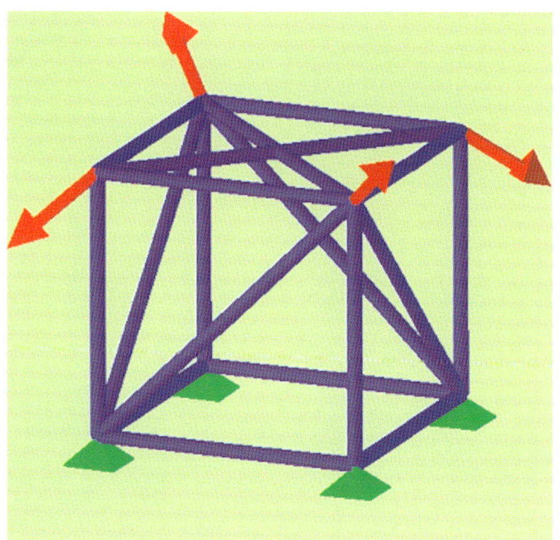

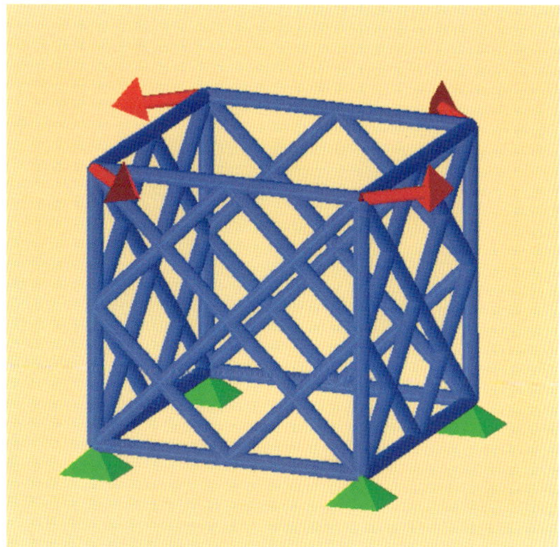

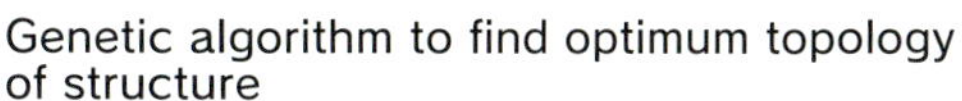

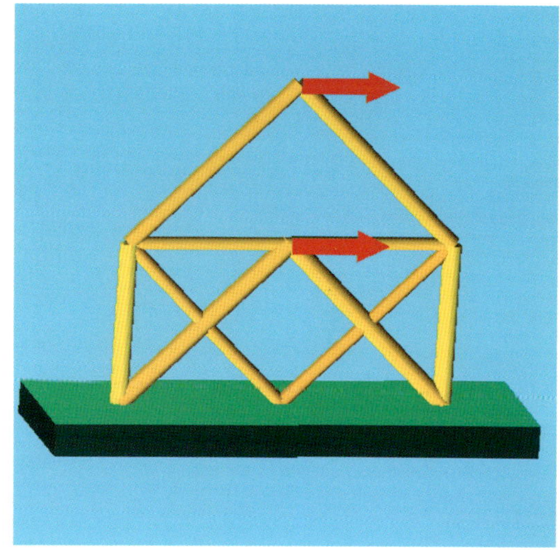

Genetic algorithm to find optimum topology of structure

The genetic algorithm arises from the theory of evolution based on the survival of the fittest. We can find the optimum topology of structural stiffness by employing the genetic algorithm. The algorithm seems valid for structural design, even though the survival of the fittest is sometimes criticized as the theory of imperialism.

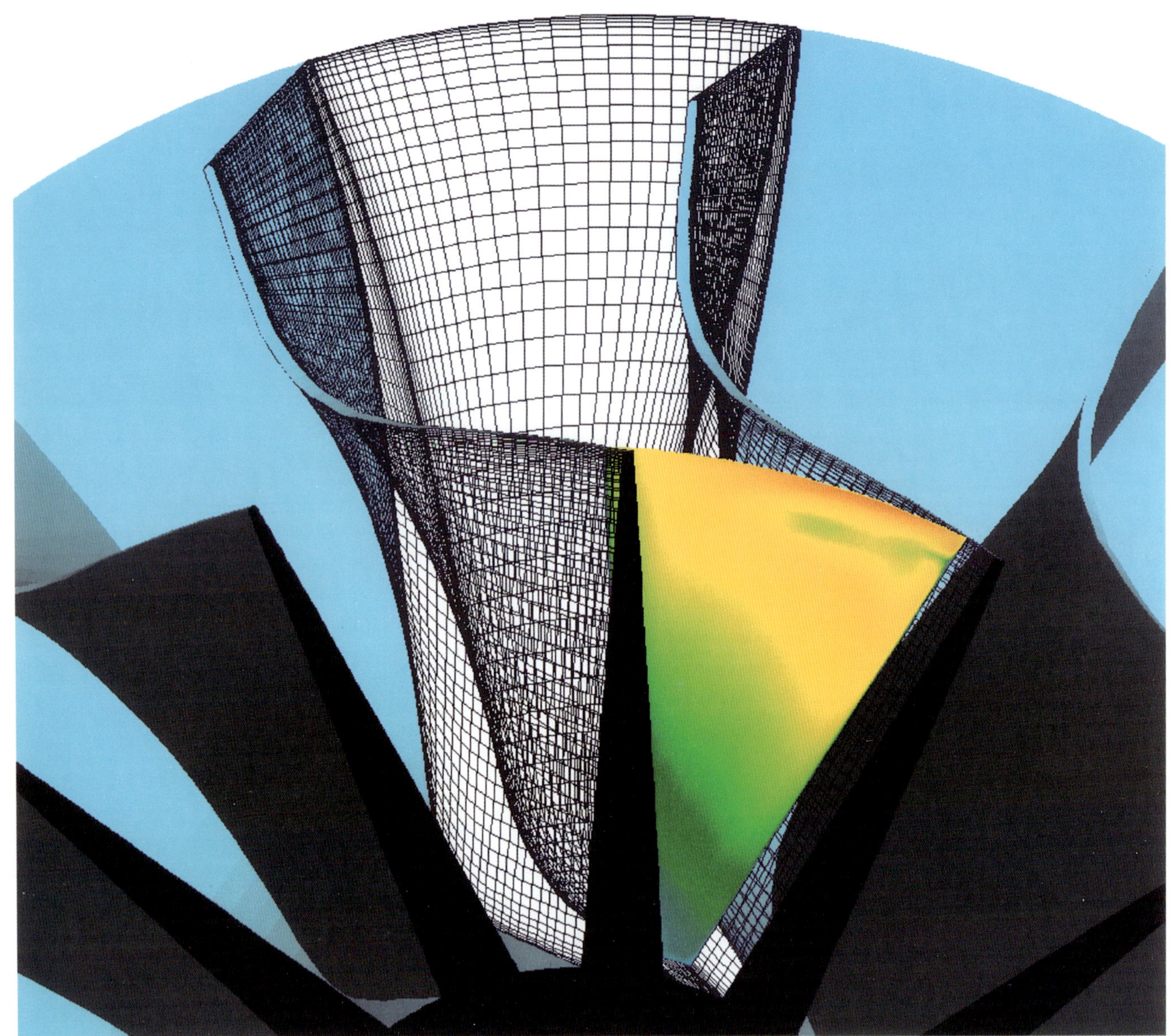

3-D flow analysis in radial turbine rotor passage

Radial turbines are widely used as turbochargers and small gas turbines. 3-D flow analysis has been performed in a radial turbine rotor with tip clearance in order to clarify the structure of losses due to secondary flow and tip leakage flow in rotor passages, and to propose a new design concept of radial turbines with high performance. The figure shows distributions of relative velocity magnitude at rotor exit.

Simulation of temperature variation in a heat pipe

The figure shows a series of numerical results of the temperature distribution in a meandering closed-loop heat pipe. White parts correspond to vapor while colored parts correspond to liquid columns. Numerical simulation gives useful information for systems where it is difficult to measure the temperature distribution.

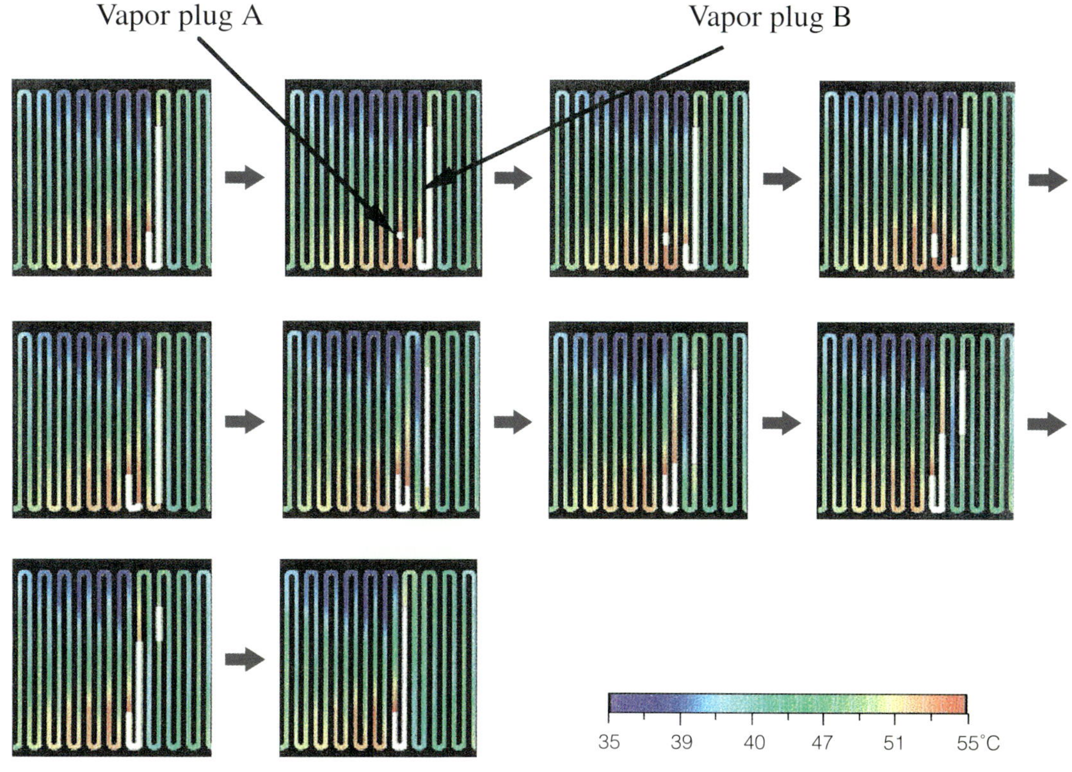

Finite element simulation system for the visualization of internal stress and plastic deformation in metal forming

Large-scale FEM simulation is now being used practically in the field of steel rolling. Rolling theory, which has been investigated over 70 years, is undergoing very rapid innovation with the help of three-dimensional deformation analysis using FEM simulation. Now FEM simulation is regarded as a key technology for the steel rolling industry.

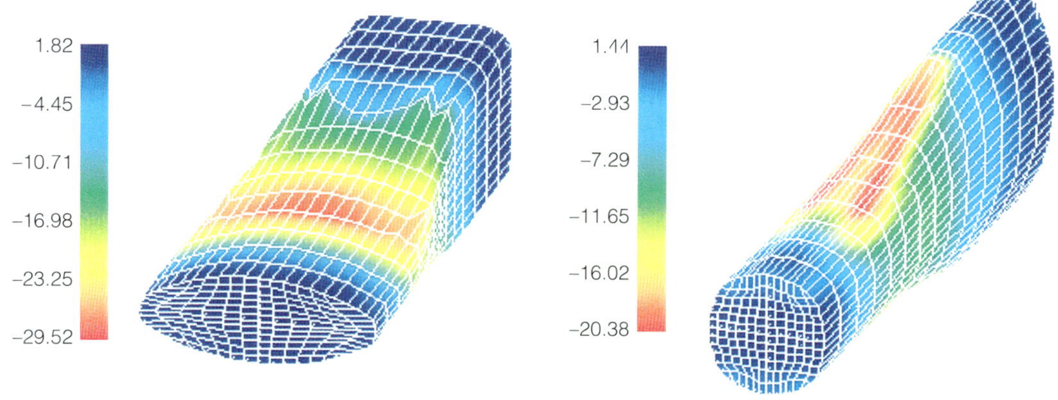

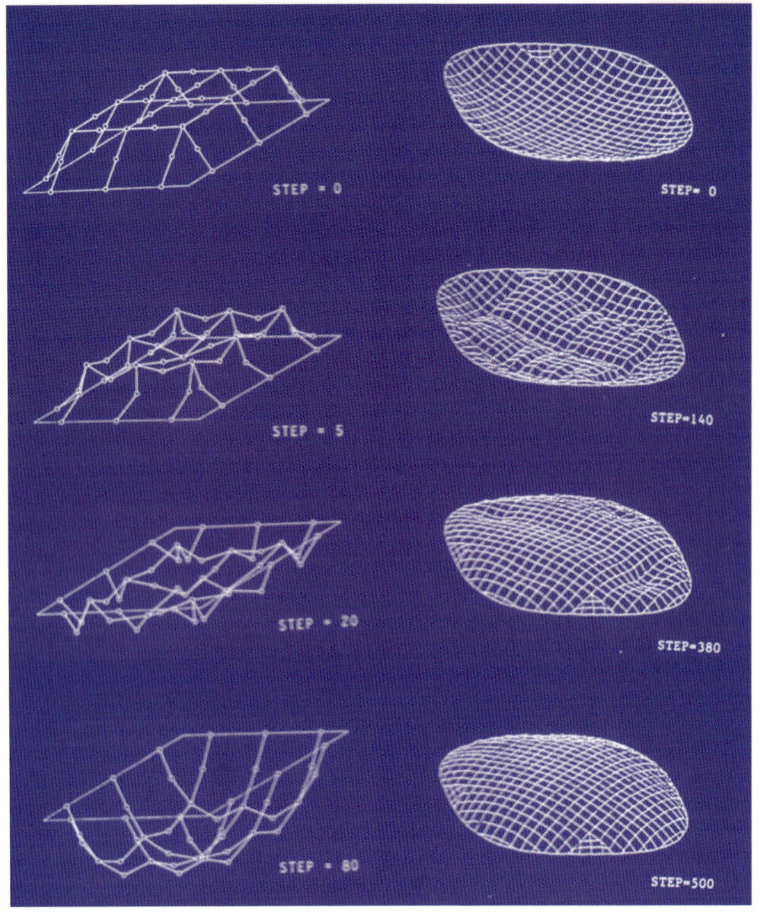

Research of lightweight flexible structures

Demands for large enclosures such as sport halls, exhibition centers and baseball stadia are increasing. Furthermore, larger covered spaces seem to be required. Shell structures, space frame structures and membrane structures are the spatial structural systems developed to answer such social requests. Flexible structures such as membrane structures and cable structures are classified as kinematically indeterminate structures, and these structures have great advantages when used for lightweight large space enclosures.

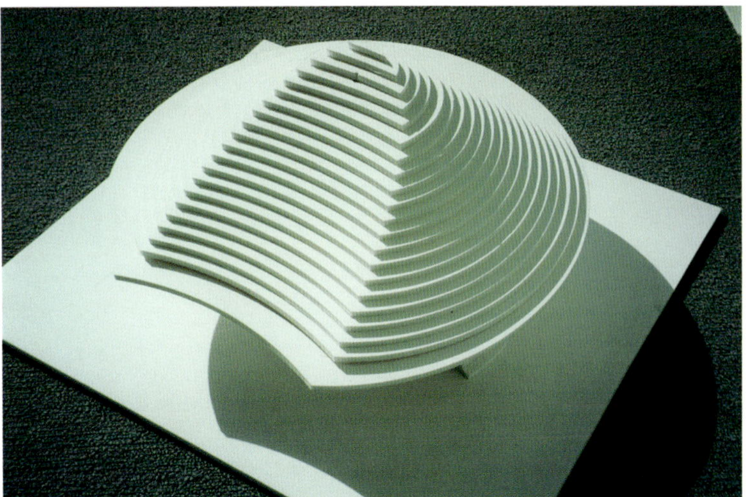

The generation of a "Topography Dome"

A new dome system, named "Topography Dome" (contour accumulation shell) is a three-dimensional architectural system with natural shape obtained by a shape generation technique (homotopy technique) based on a group of parallel closed curves. The properties of this system are as follows : 1. Form resistance structural system with natural form, 2. Higher earthquake-resistant and wind-resistant capacities, 3. Adaptability for large spaces without columns and with an arbitrary plan configuration.

Lightweight architectures with large spaces are problematic. In order to meet the future demands for larger spaces such as in a convention center or an indoor stadium, novel structure systems are being studied.

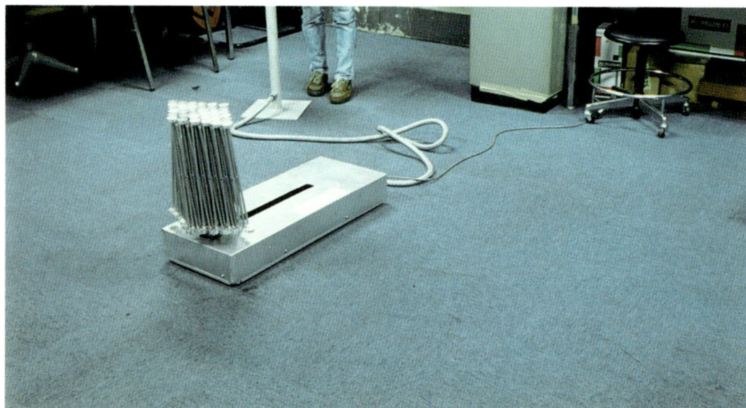

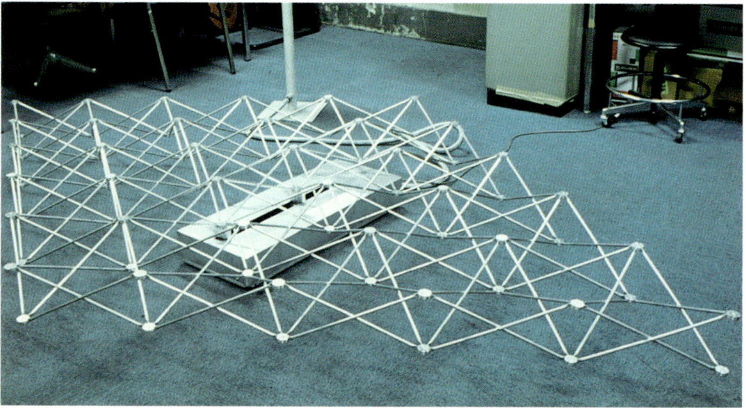

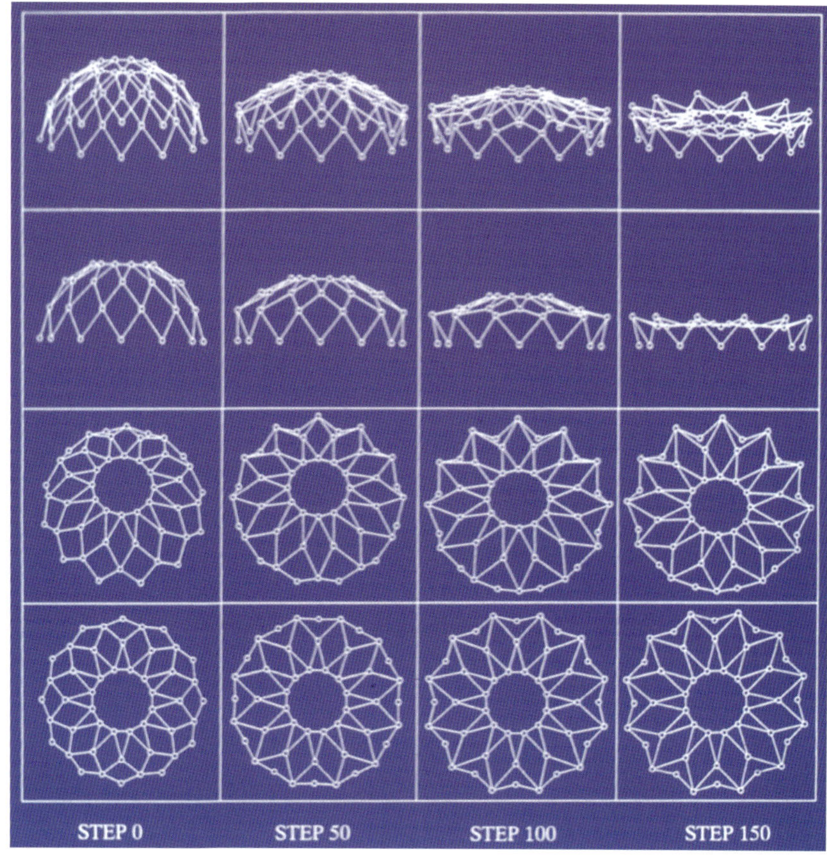

Research of deployable structures
— Analysis of folding structures

In order to build large structures in extraterrestrial space, the effective use of the limited transportation space in a space ship is important. The structure must be prepared for easy assembly. Such structures are usually designed as deployable structures that can be folded and transported compactly, and then unfolded largely ready for use. For terrestrial structures, folding structures can also have great advantages in transportation and construction.

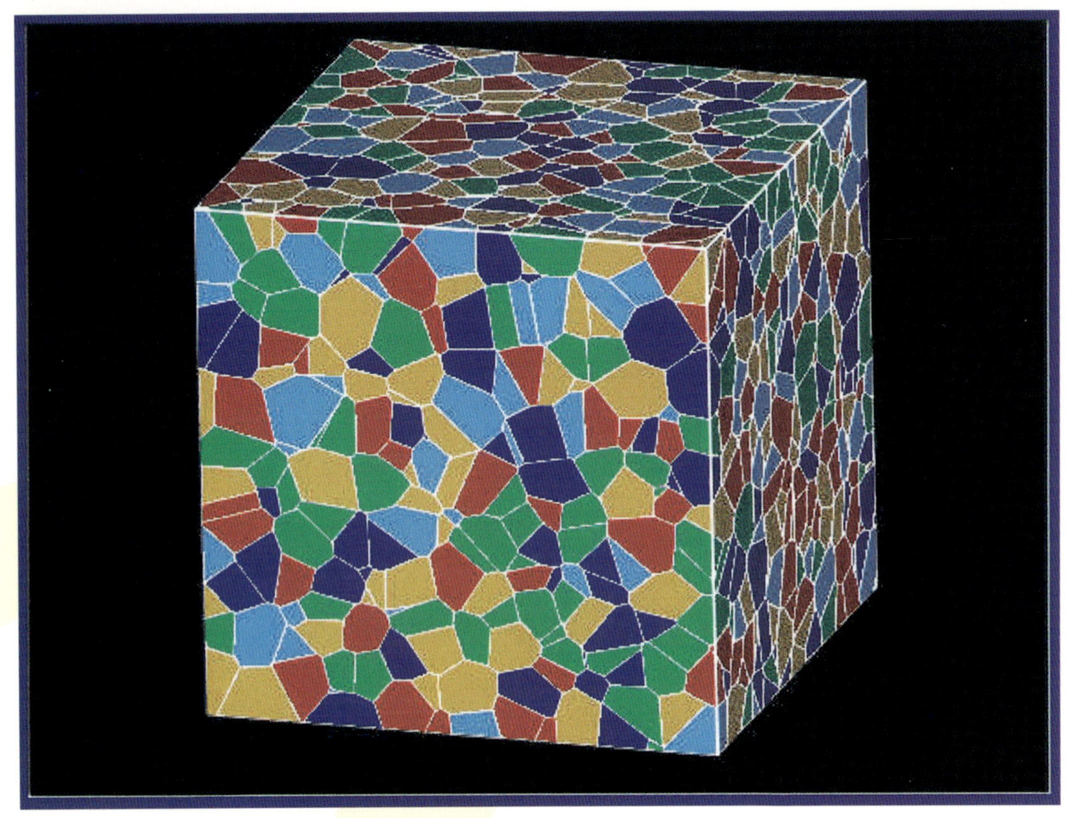

Mesoscopic simulation of brittle microcracking solids

It is indispensable to the design of machines and structures to solve the internal damage and fracture behavior of brittle microcracking solids such as ceramic materials under mechanical loading. The figure shows a model to simulate the microcracking behavior of brittle polycrystalline solids at a mesoscopic scale (grain scale) which is composed of about 3,400 crystal grains.

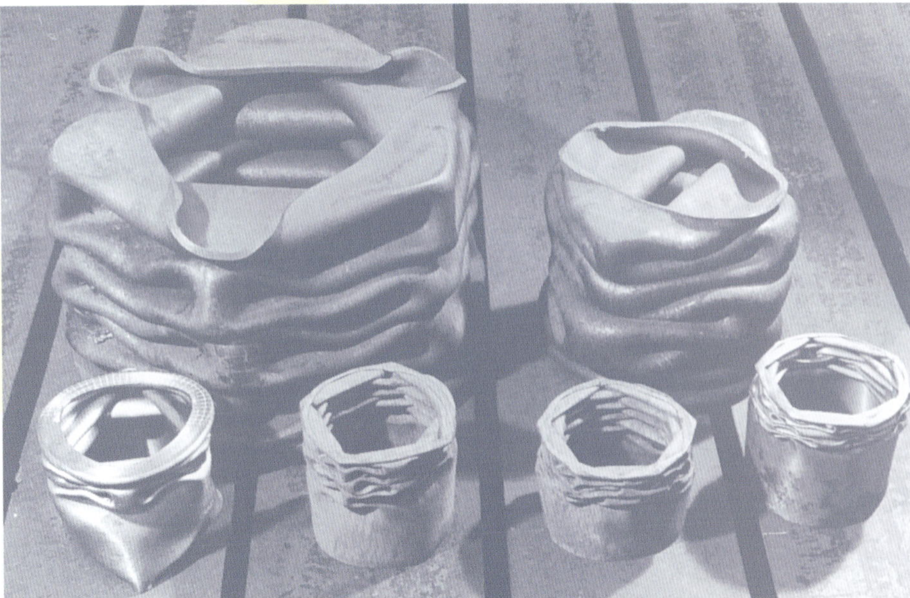

Crushing deformation of circular tubes

Interesting shapes are observed in the crushing deformation of circular steel tubes under axial loadings. As shown in the figure, various cross-sectional deformations are observed, such as an elliptical, triangular, square, pentagonal, or hexagonal shape. This sort of experimental data is necessary for the structural design against an extremely large loading such as a collision.

Crush analysis of square tubes

Extremely severe loading such as a collision causes structural crush, which is a highly nonlinear problem accompanied by large displacement, large strains and frictional contact. The figure shows the result for axial crushing of a square tube analyzed by the finite element method, which is utilized in the design of crashworthiness of automobile body structures.

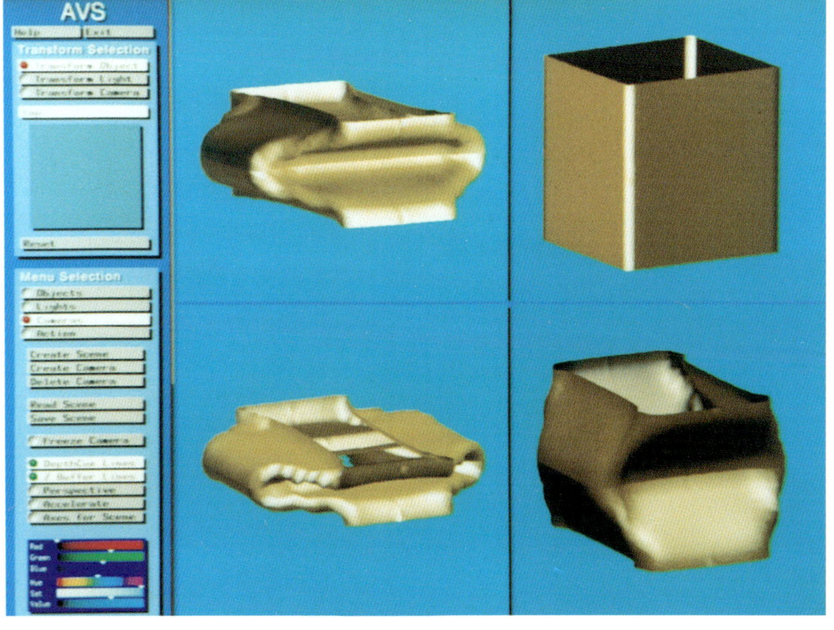

Simulation of fracture behaviors of two-phase materials

The internal cracking behaviour of a two-phase material composed of a bulk material (such as alumina) and second-phase particles (such as zirconia), can be simulated by the method of mesoscopic analysis at a grain scale. This elucidates the effect of mechanical properties of the bulk material, the particles, and their interface on the overall fracture strength.

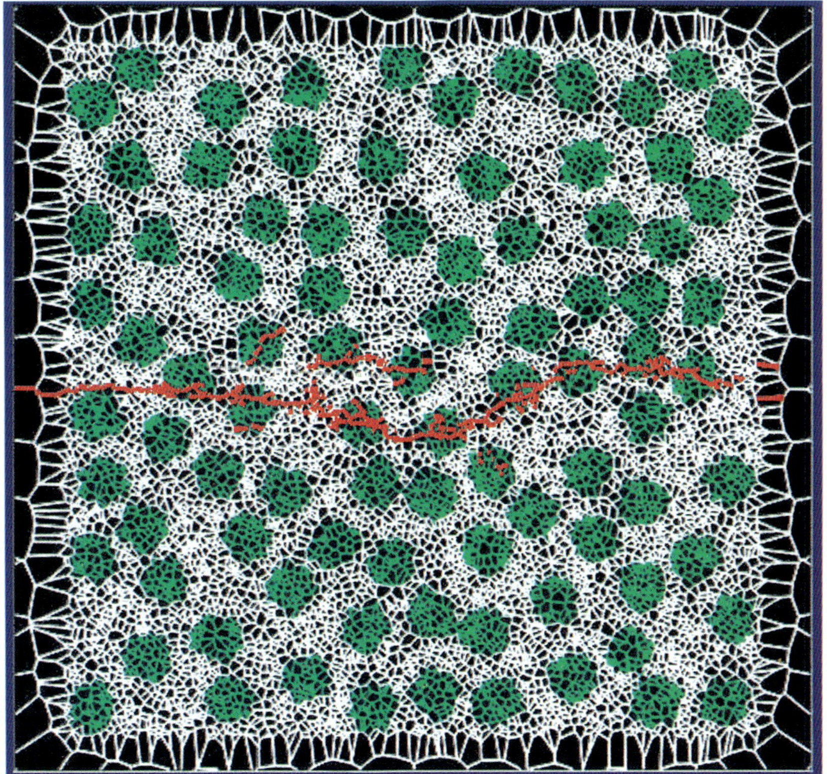

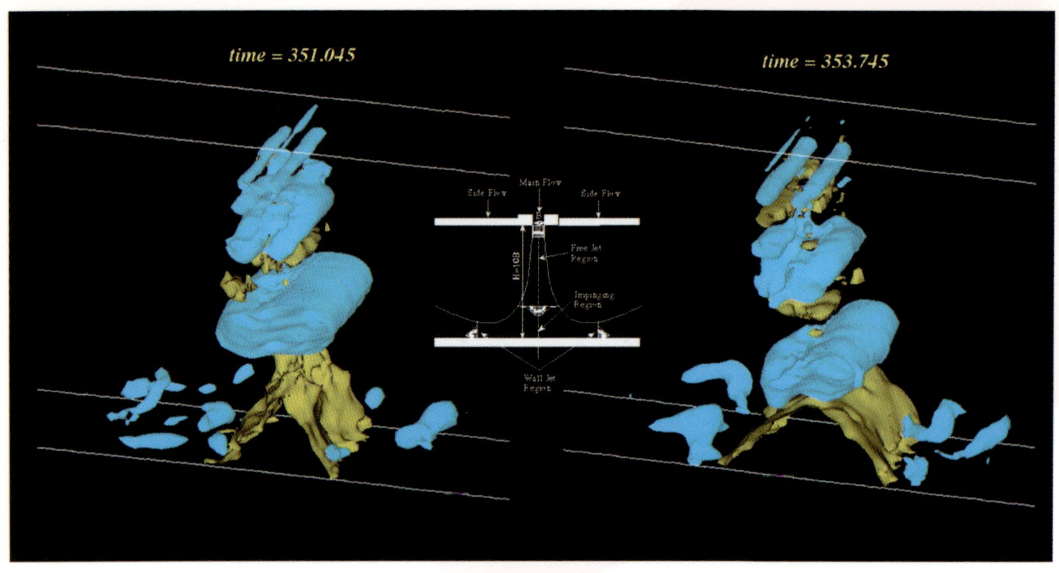

LES of a plane impinging jet

An impinging jet is one of the fundamental flow structures, and is dealt with in various industrial applications such as chemical processing. Large Eddy Simulation (LES) makes it feasible to investigate organized structures in three dimensions. The figure shows instantaneous pressure iso-surface of the plane impinging jet at two different elapsed times as results of LES. The pressure field is almost two-dimensional near the nozzle exit region. However, after the impinging, LES describes a fully 3-D structure.

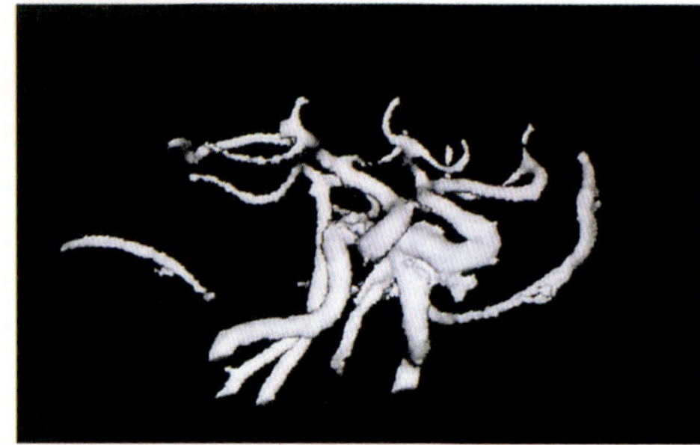

The internal carotid artery

Velocity vectors in the center plane

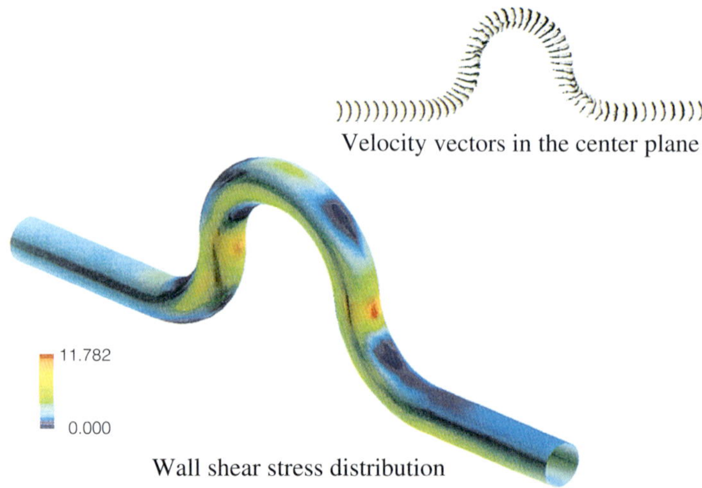

Wall shear stress distribution

Numerical simulation of a blood flow in the internal carotid artery

Numerical simulation has increasingly become one of the important applications in the medical field. The medical study shows that an aneurysm occurs mostly around a bifurcation area in the internal carotid with large curvature, and the geometry of the blood vessel changes according to age and sex. The figure shows the wall shear stress and the velocity vector as a result of the simplified numerical model of the internal carotid artery as a curved blood vessel to examine an effect due to curvature. The result shows the periodic oscillations in the flow field.

LES of turbulent flow around a stationary and oscillating rectangular cylinder

The geometry of a turbulent flow around a rectangular cylinder is rather simple although it features complicated flow structures. In order to capture transient 3-D structures of the flow, the LES is used to simulate turbulent flow around a stationary and oscillating rectangular cylinder. The formation of the Kármán vortex street with fluctuations is clearly observed and the flow behind the rectangular cylinder is fully three-dimensional.

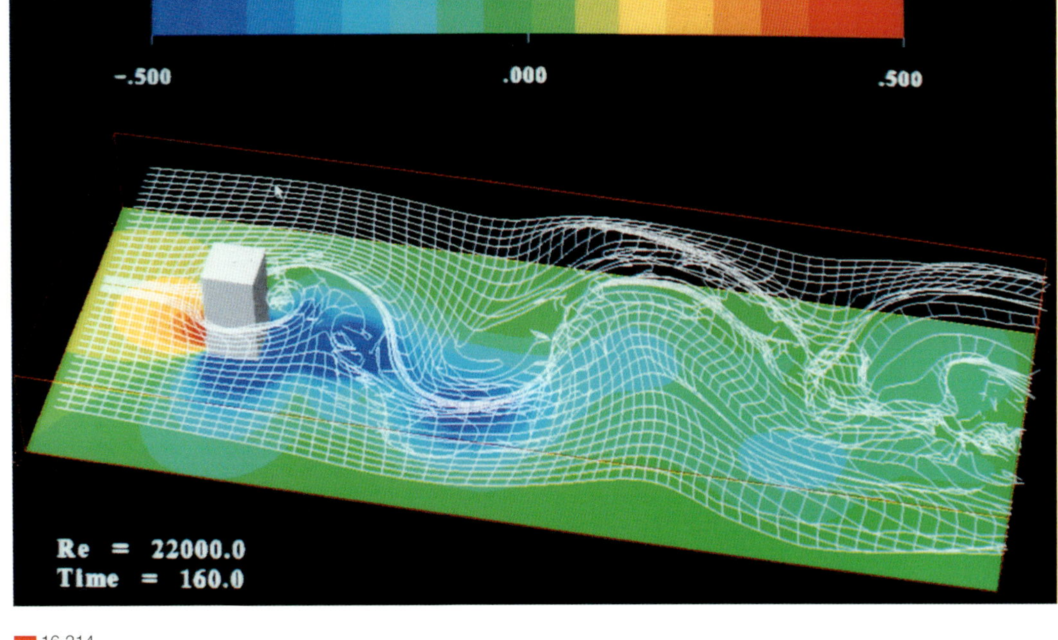

LES of turbulent flow in a combustion device

The flow with chemical reactions is an important industrial application. It is important to estimate precisely the turbulent mixing process since the turbulent mixing rate is a key factor to designing the gas turbine combustor. In the context of energy efficiency, it is also necessary to optimize the promotion of the turbulent mixing process for a flame holder. All these features depend on the accurate prediction of a turbulent flow field. The figure shows instantaneous vorticity distribution behind the flame holder predicted by the LES. It describes the process of production and destruction of two ring-shape vortexes generated behind the flame holder.

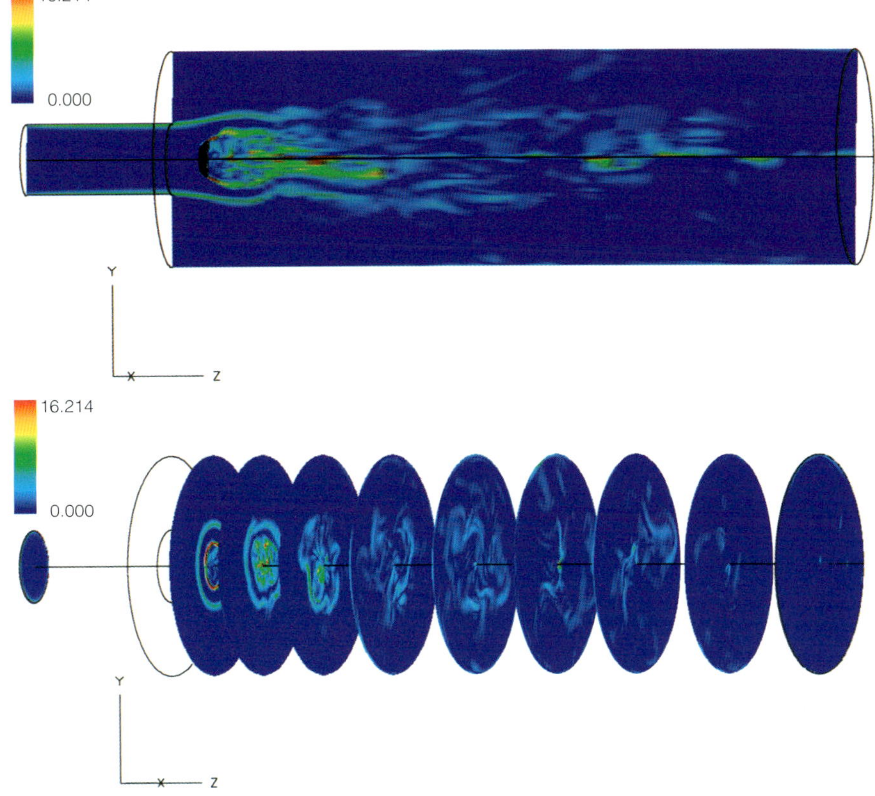

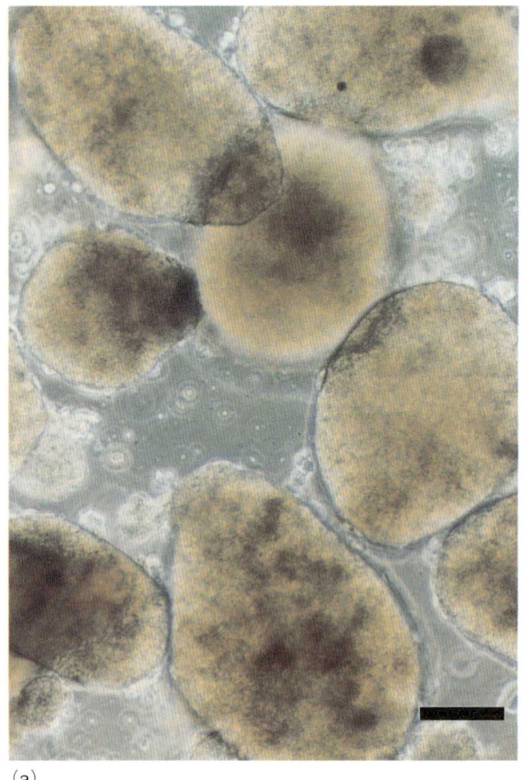

(a)

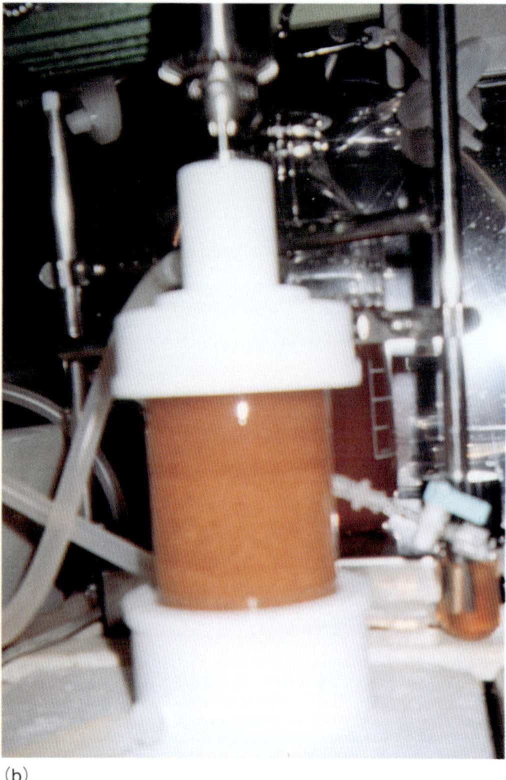

(b)

Reconstituted liver tissue and it's application to bio-artificial livers

Designing compact and high-performance bio-reactors is one of the crucial issues in developing bio-artificial liver systems for the treatment of patients with acute liver failure. The photographs show the morphology of pig liver tissues reconstituted in vitro (spheroids, fig. (a), bar=100 μm) and a compact bio-reactor based on high-cell density suspension perfusion culture of such spheroids (fig. (b)). This bio-reactor design allows the spheroids to express their maximal metabolic activities due to its good mass transfer between the spheroids and the perfused patient's plasma.

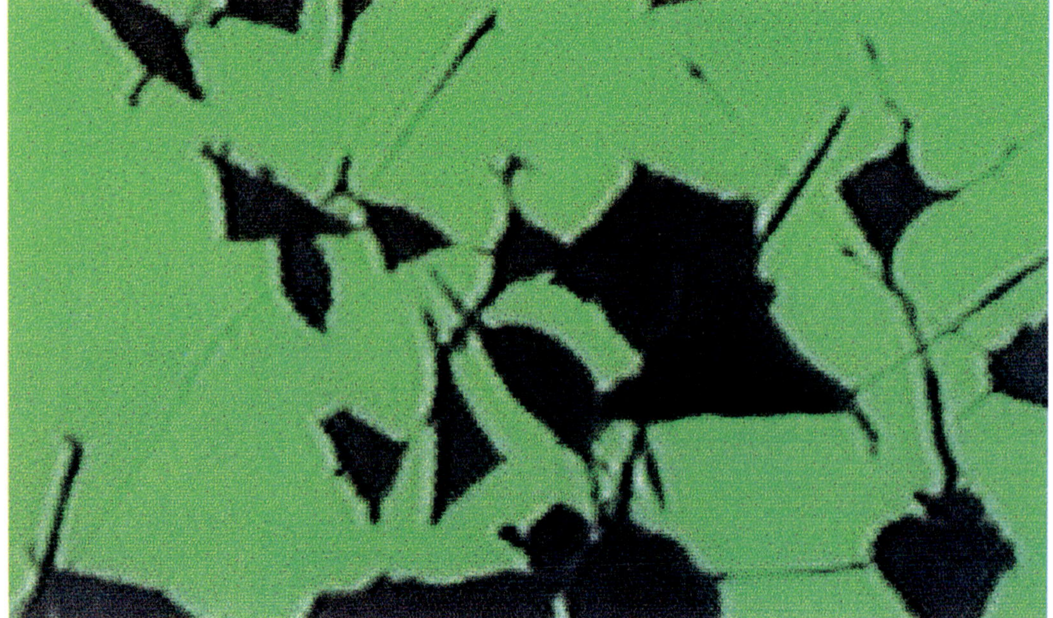

Attempts to evaluate toxity of water using cultured mammalian cells

For proper risk assessment and management of toxic chemicals in the near future, simple methodologies for toxicity evaluation systems using cultured mammalian cells are expected to become standard procedures. We have developed this kind of simple assay based on cell growth, functional deterioration or morphological changes of various mammalian cells. The photograph shows a stained image of cultured nerve cells. We can evaluate the neuro-specific toxicity of environmental pollutants by the changes in the nerve fiber length.

Proposed mechanism for inhibition of HIV by curdlan sulfate and its detection by NMR

Anti-HIV activity displayed by curdlan sulfated poly-and oligo-saccharides with high anti-HIV activity were investigated. Curdlan sulfate having strong anti-HIV and protozoan activity, and sulfated alkyl oligo-saccharids were synthesized. In order to elucidate the mechanism of high anti-HIV activity, NMR analyses were carried out by using an HIV protein model and curdlan sulfate. It was found that there were significant interactions between cations of protein and anions of sulfated saccharides.

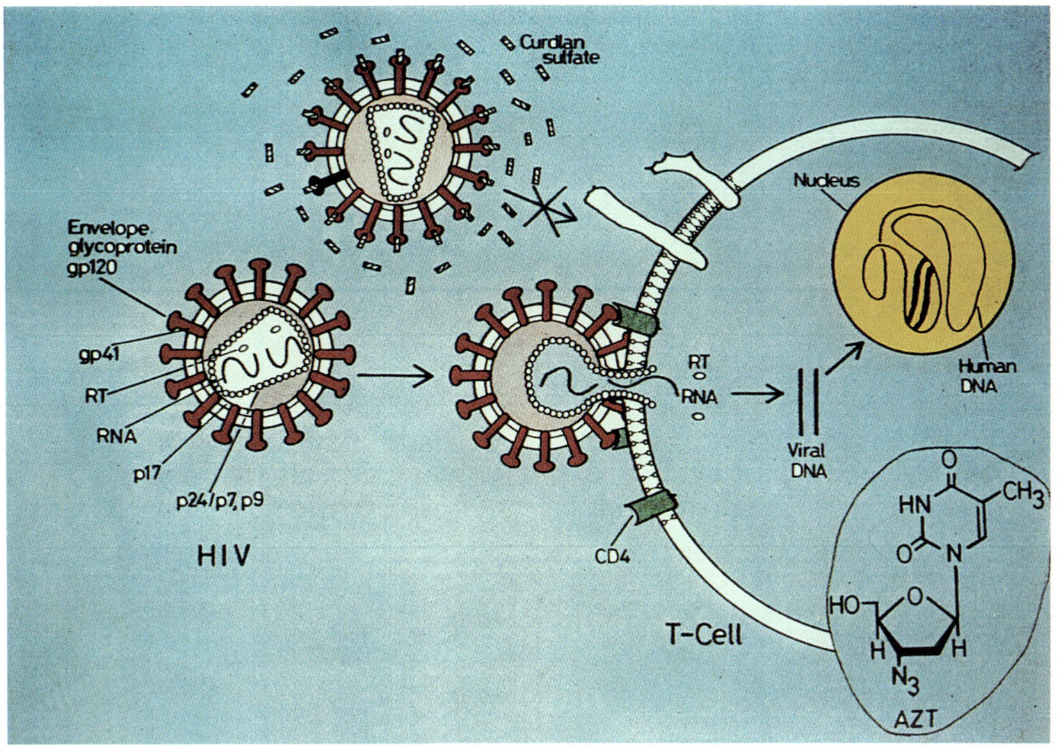

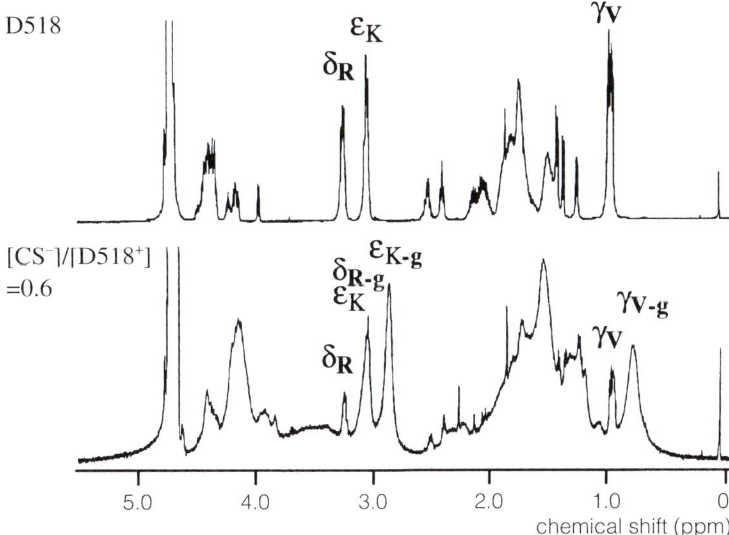

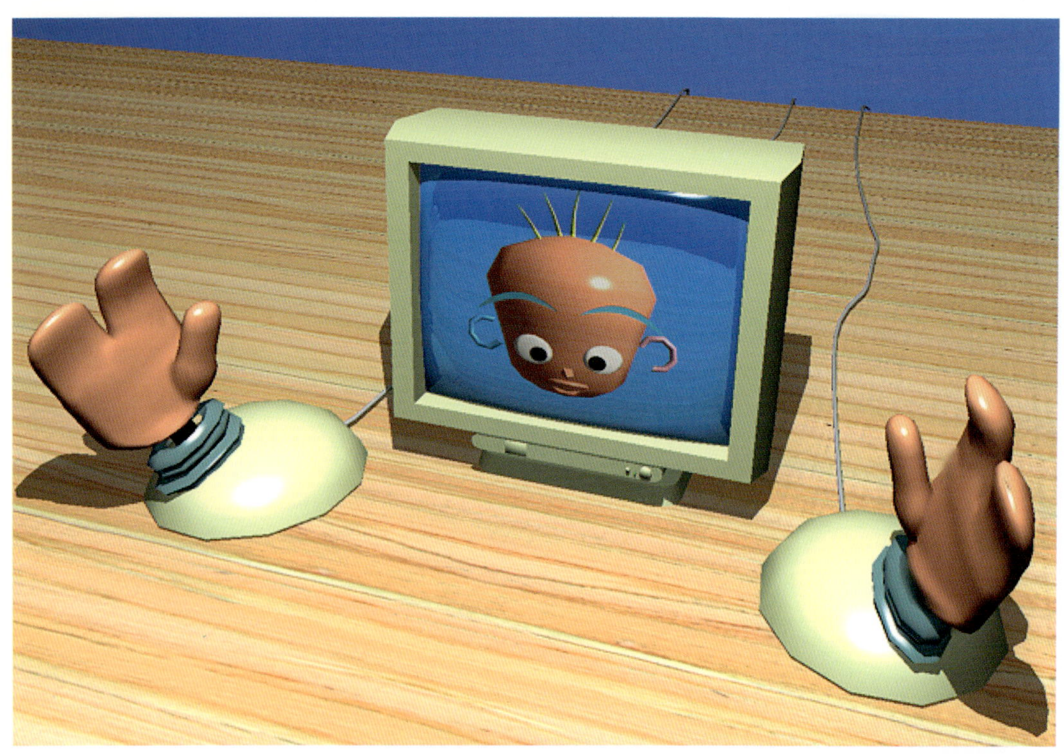

An experiment of non-verbal communication

A computer agent which simulates the emotions and behaviors of a baby was set up on a site in Japan and in the USA. Along with these, a hand-shaking device with which the force of handshake can be transmitted was also set up. Using these, we studied the possibility of non-verbal communication. Although it was an awkward experiment, it was verified that the transmission of certain concepts is possible.

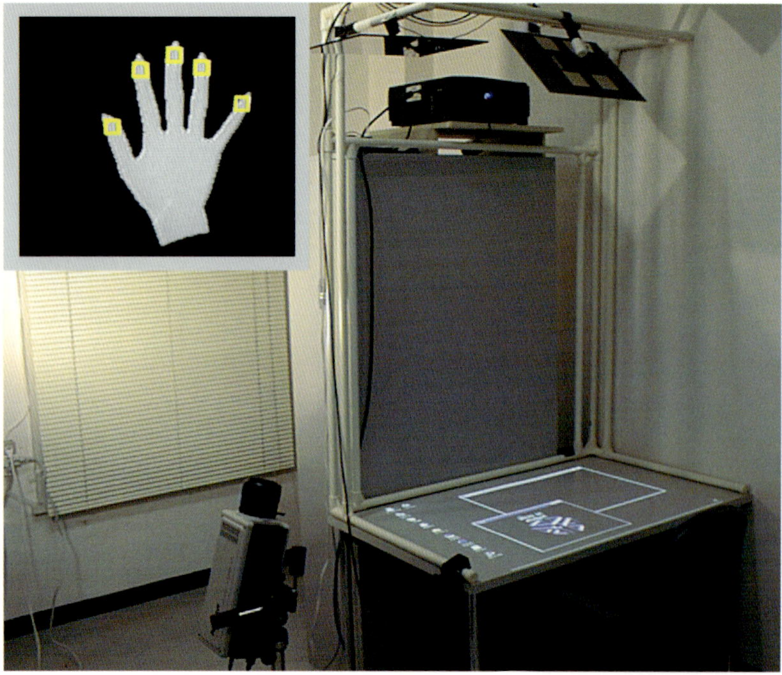

Enhanced desktop environment

In this project, we have been investigating a novel form of human-computer interaction. In particular, users are allowed to explore both physical information stored in papers or books, and digital information retrieved from computer networks, without feeling any gaps between them. To achieve such human-computer interaction, real-time computer vision technologies play a fundamental role in understanding the user's motions (e.g., hand gestures and gaze directions) in real-time without using any invasive devices.

Appearance modeling for mixed reality

Mixed reality allows a user to see the real world with virtual objects superimposed, while virtual reality technologies completely immerse a user inside a synthetic environment. Our efforts on mixed reality cover two aspects: how to create models of virtual objects, and how to integrate such virtual objects with the real world. By analyzing the physical properties of real object surfaces and the illumination of the real world, we can accomplish high-quality presentations of mixed reality environments.

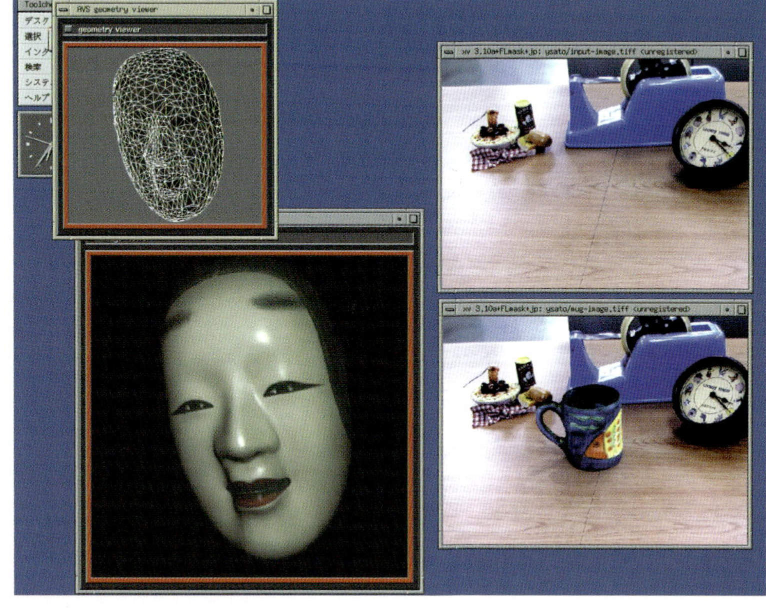

Assembly plan from observation

Currently, robot programming is done either by manual programming or by the "teaching-by-showing" method using a teach pendant. Both methods have been found to have several drawbacks. We have been developing a novel method of programming a robot, the Assembly-Plan-from-Observation (APO) method. The APO system observes a human performing an assembly task, understands it, and generates a robot program to achieve that same assembly task.

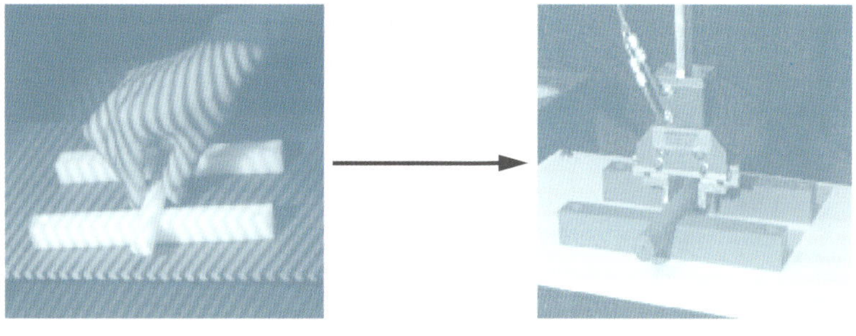

Modeling from reality

We are developing techniques to construct solid models from observation of real objects. Research projects include: building a virtual corridor of the I.I.S. building using a moveable range-finder cart; building human busts from a sequence of images; and building appearance models for vision algorithm compiler.

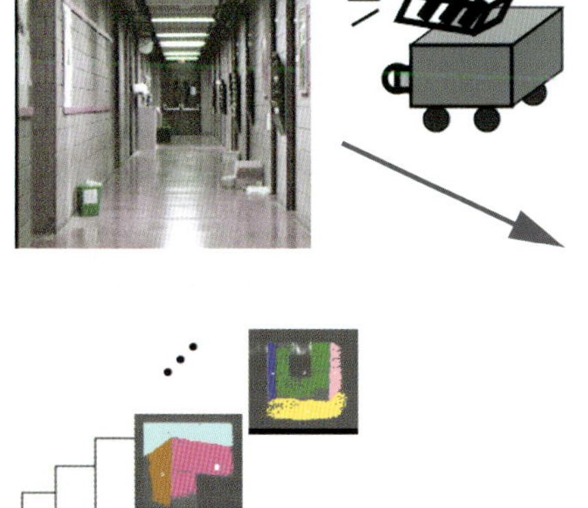

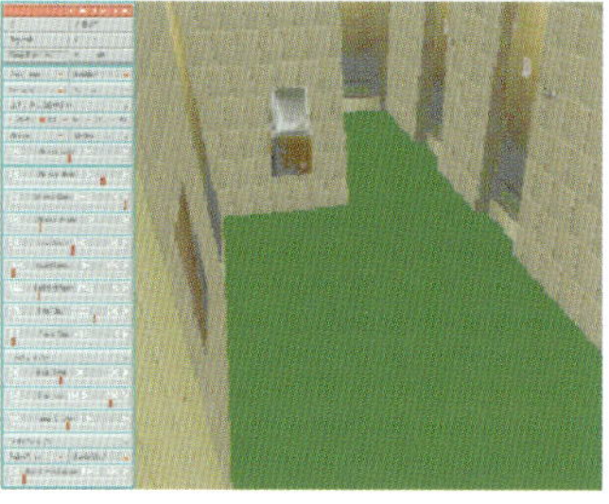

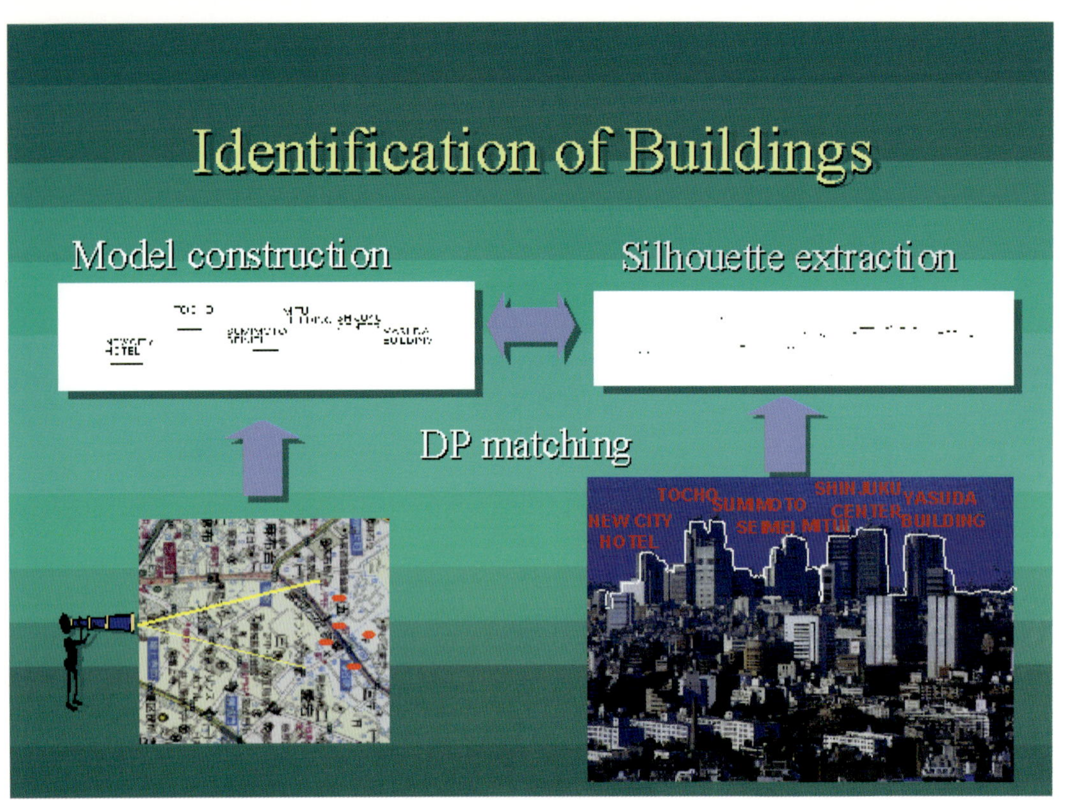

Recognition of urban scenes in distant views

We proposed an approach for understanding urban scenes in distant views by recognizing key buildings, which appear as silhouettes using model-based object recognition. The figure shows the locating results based on the correspondence between the silhouettes and a 3-model obtained from a map.

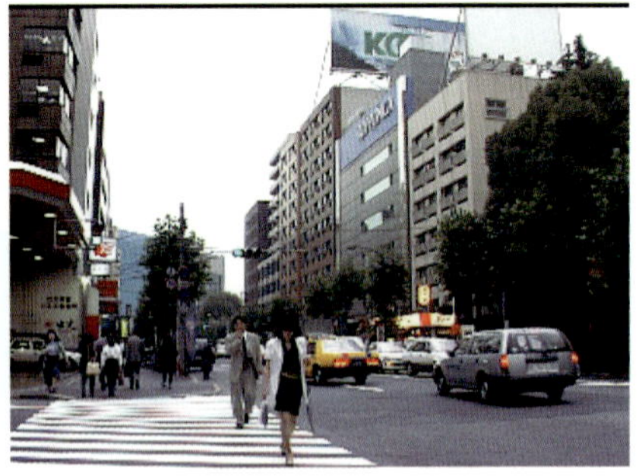
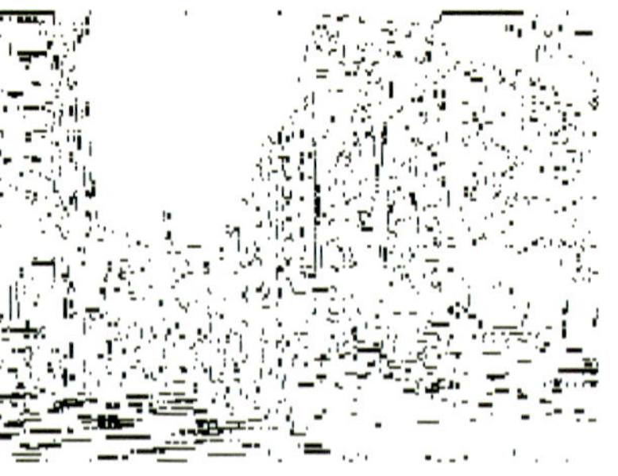
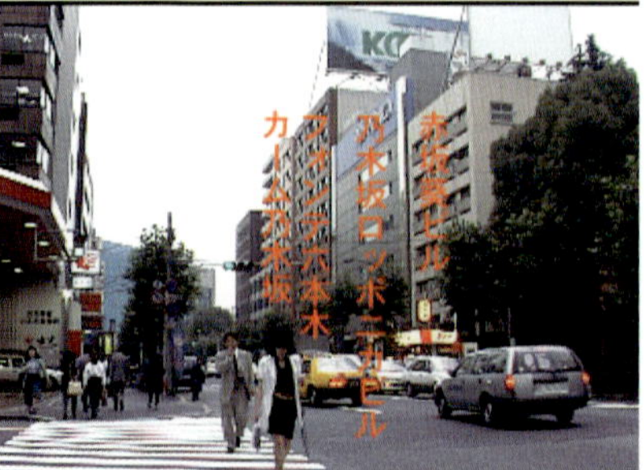

Recognition of urban scenes in close-range views

Recognizing urban scenes in close-range views is another part of our research. The eigen space and database technique is applied to recognize urban scenes in close-range views. The figure shows the results of building identification.

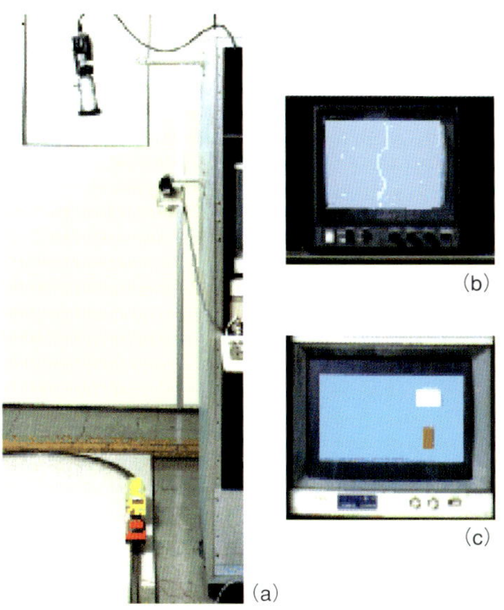

(b)

(c)

(a)

Vehicle detection using laser-beam cutting method

We have developed a novel image sensor for measuring not only the number of vehicles but also their velocity and size. The laser beam is spread onto the road like a curtain, along the center of a lane. The observed beam looks like several lines (top right figure) and we can calculate the height and the velocity of vehicles.

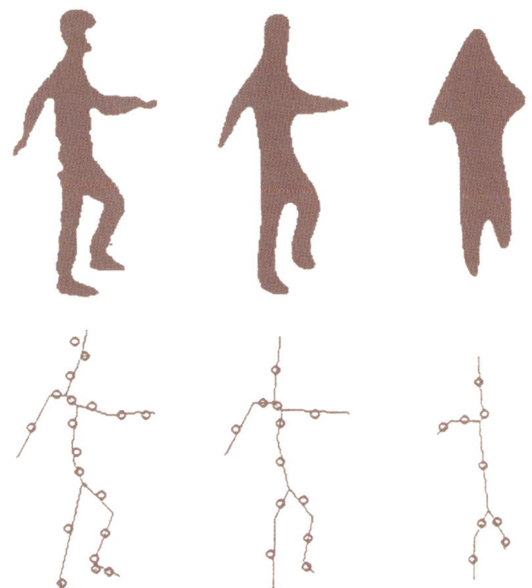

Description of shape by sequentially smoothing outline

Top figures : Silhouettes of a walker whose outlines are smoothed to varying degrees. Bottom figures : "Skeletons" of the corresponding silhouettes. Based on the relationships between the skeletons, the shape of an image region is described in a hierarchical way. From this descriptive data, various approximate shapes can be reconstructed efficiently.

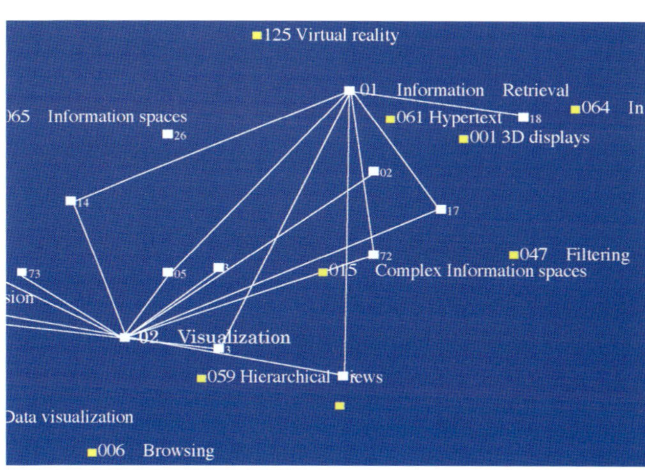

Interactive visualization of document space

We have developed a visual interaction technique to explore a large collection of documents. Documents and keywords are laid out dynamically in order to compose a semantic map of the document space. Manipulating these visualized items, the user can arrange the layout of the map according to his or her viewpoint.

(a)

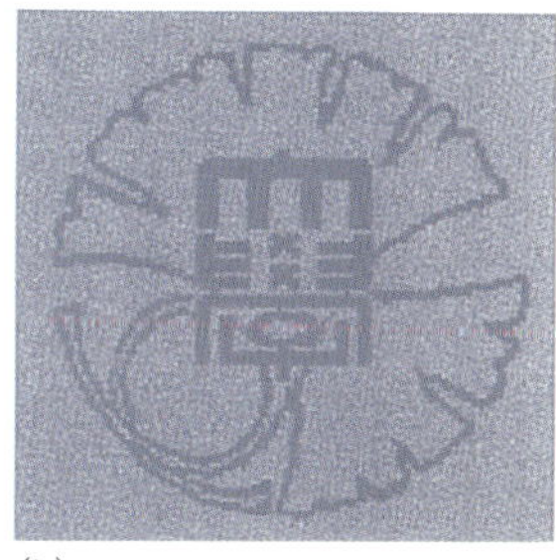

(b)

Visual secret sharing schemes

The image (fig. (a)) is divided into 3 random-like patterns (fig. (b)) by using a visual secret sharing scheme. The original image can then be decoded by stacking any 2 of the patterns. Such techniques are useful in managing very important information among some members.

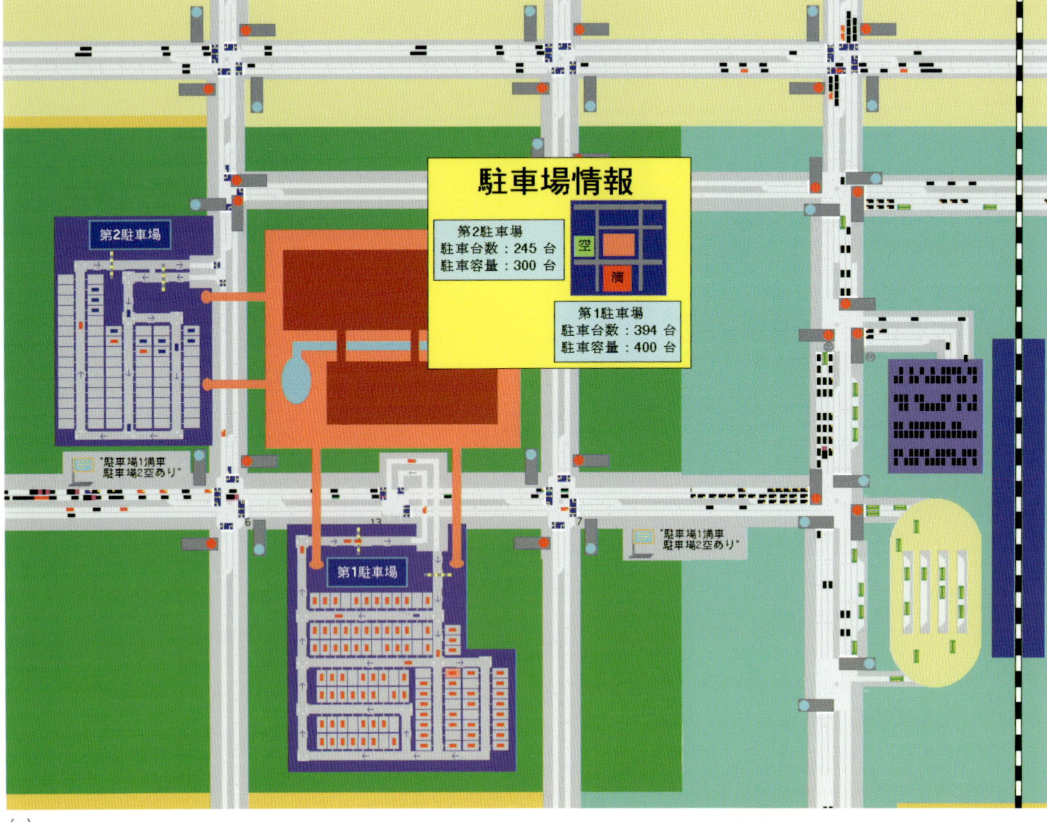

(a)

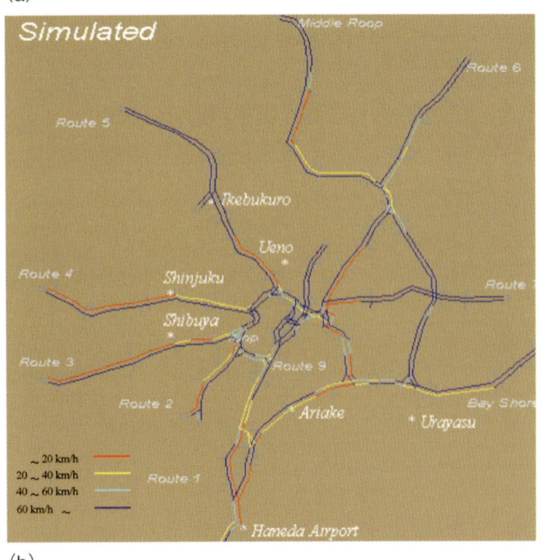

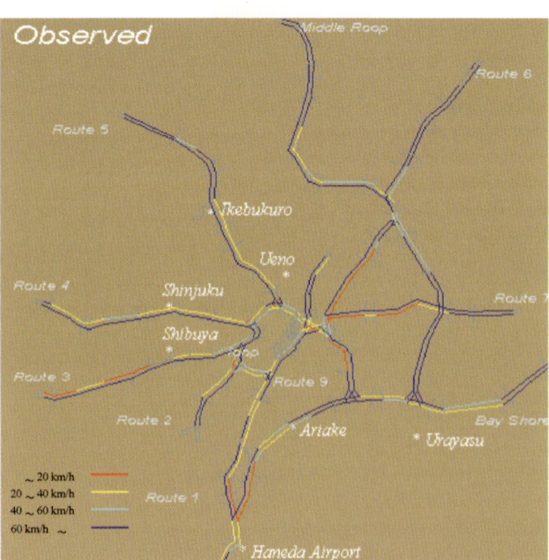

(b)

Traffic simulation models for urban networks — SOUND and AVENUE

SOUND and AVENUE are network simulation models developed in the Kuwahara lab. SOUND can handle a large network with thousands of links and nodes, while AVENUE deals with a relatively small network but reproduces traffic conditions in a more detailed way under various signal control strategies and traffic regulations.

It is essential to predict and control human flow in order to smooth human activities in contemporary overcrowded cities. Here, let us introduce examples of predictions of human activity in a city.

New philosophy of safety design for urban spaces, from the viewpoint of human evacuation

To build safe city spaces and structures, as well ensuring structural strength, it is also very important to ensure the safety of the users in both normal and emergency situations. We have developed a new evacuation model in which the individual personality of the users, the effects of a disaster such as smoke and fire, and also the effects of evacuation guidance can all be consider-ed. Using this model, the safety of the spaces and the efficiency of evacuation guidance can be evaluated.

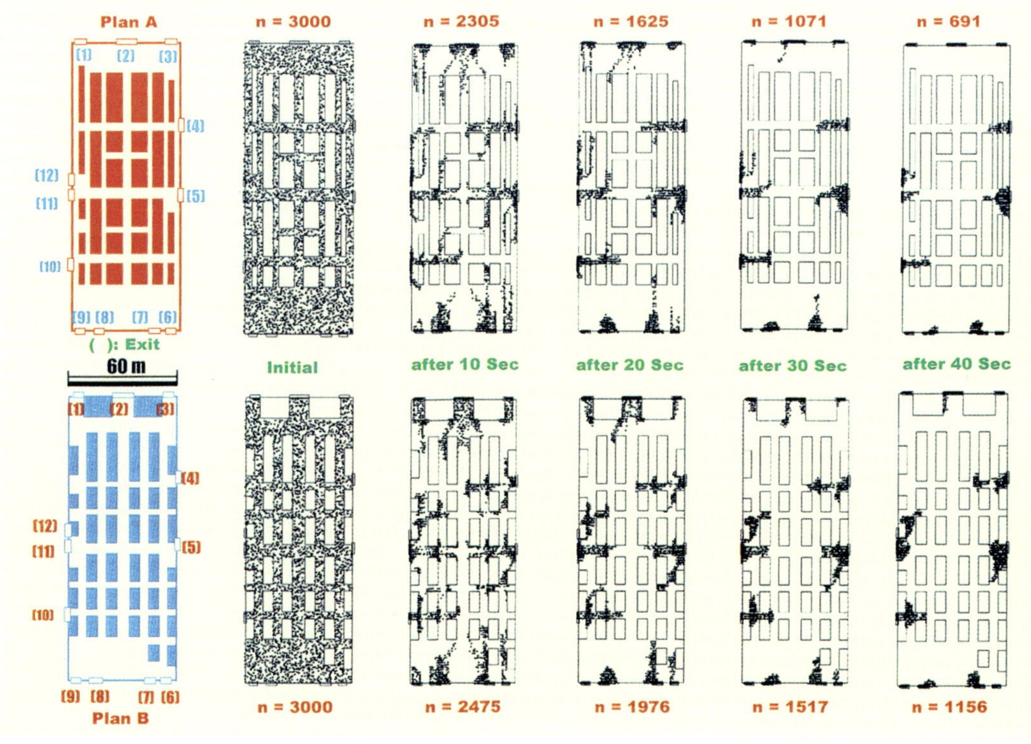

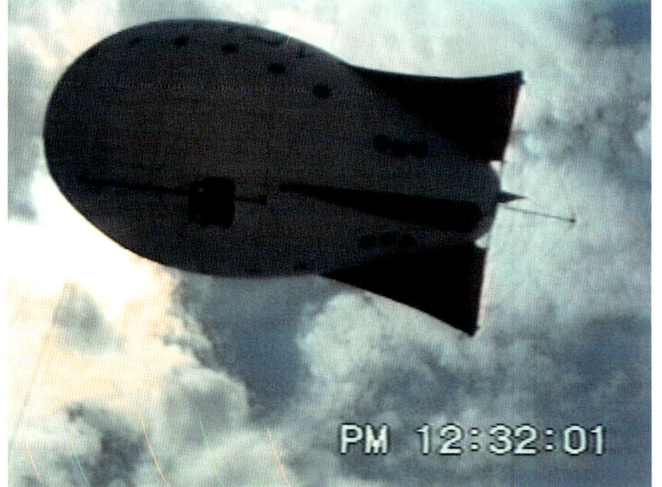

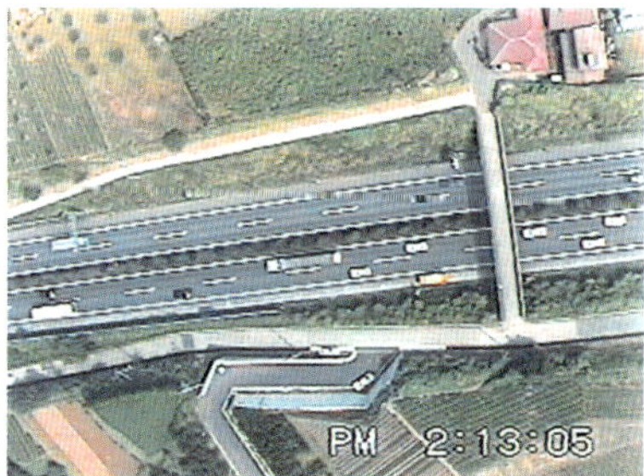

An observation system of vehicle motion

An automatic vehicle tracking system from video images has been developed, and it processes video images taken for example from an observa-tion halloon. An experimental vehicle has been also made in order to observe vehicle motion : the velocity, acceleration, headway and other parameters. These data sources are utilized to analyze highway capacity, developing simulation models, and so on.

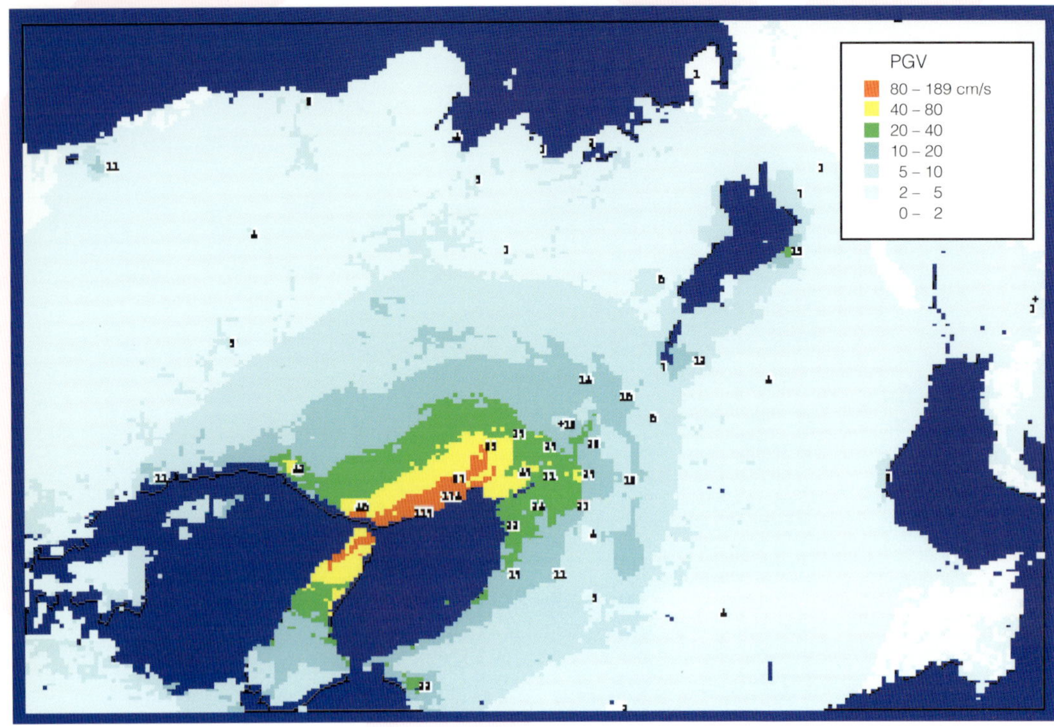

Distribution of estimated PGV in the 1995 Hyogoken-Nanbu Earthquake

Using strong motion records obtained by newly-installed seismic networks, attenuation relations were developed for the Peak Ground Acceleration (PGA), Peak Ground Velocity (PGV), response spectra and the instrumental JMA intensity. The relationship between the strong ground motion indices and structural damage was investigated using the actual damage data and the results of numerical analyses. The figure indicates the estimated surface PGV in the 1995 Hyogoken-Nanbu Earthquake based on a stochastic interpolation method.

Flood inundation simulation and damage estimation from the Ichinomiya river floods, September 1996 →

A new integrated mathematical model for flood inundation simulation and damage assessment has been developed. The figure illustrates an application of the model in the Ichinomiya river basin, Chiba prefecture, Japan. The top figure shows a simulation of the flood inundation using physically based distributed hydrologic model which occurred in September 1996. The assets within the catchment area, such as commercial and private buildings, industry, and agriculture are spatially distributed utilizing detailed land cover information derived from LANDSAT satellite images. The second layer shows a classified land cover map. The third layer shows the economic damage distribution of residential buildings, expressed in terms of 1,000 yen per 50 m square grid area. Economic damage is estimated using depth-damage functions for different types of assets.

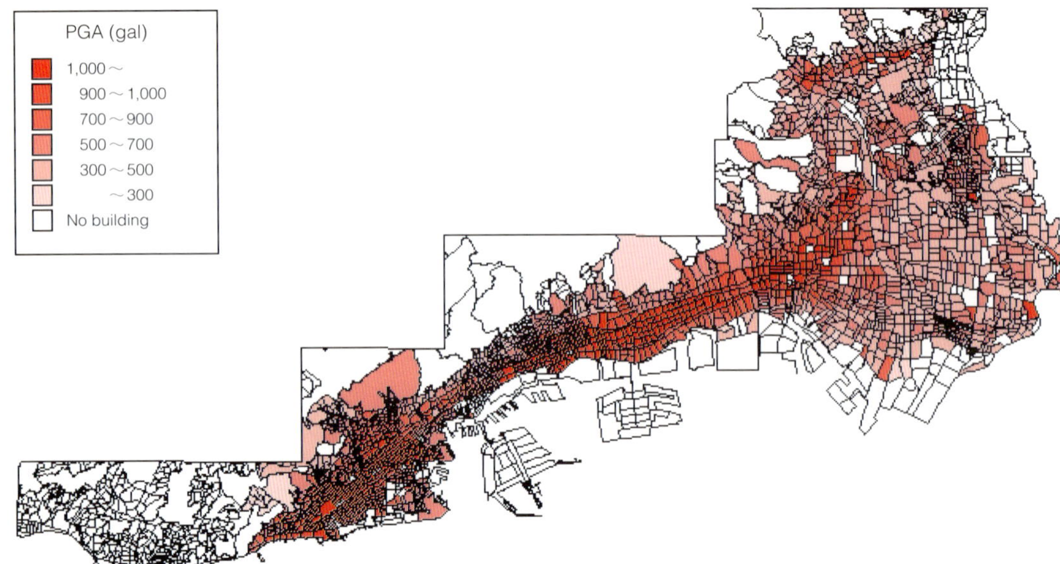

Distribution of estimated strong ground motion in the 1995 Hyogoken-Nanbu Earthquake based on building damage data

Collecting a large amount of damage survey data after the 1995 Hyogoken-Nanbu Earthquake, various correlation analyses were conducted on a Geographical Information System (GIS). The figure shows the estimated strong motion distribution (PGV) in the area hit hardest by the earthquake. Through this kind of research, we try to contribute to social seismic safety and urban safety planning.

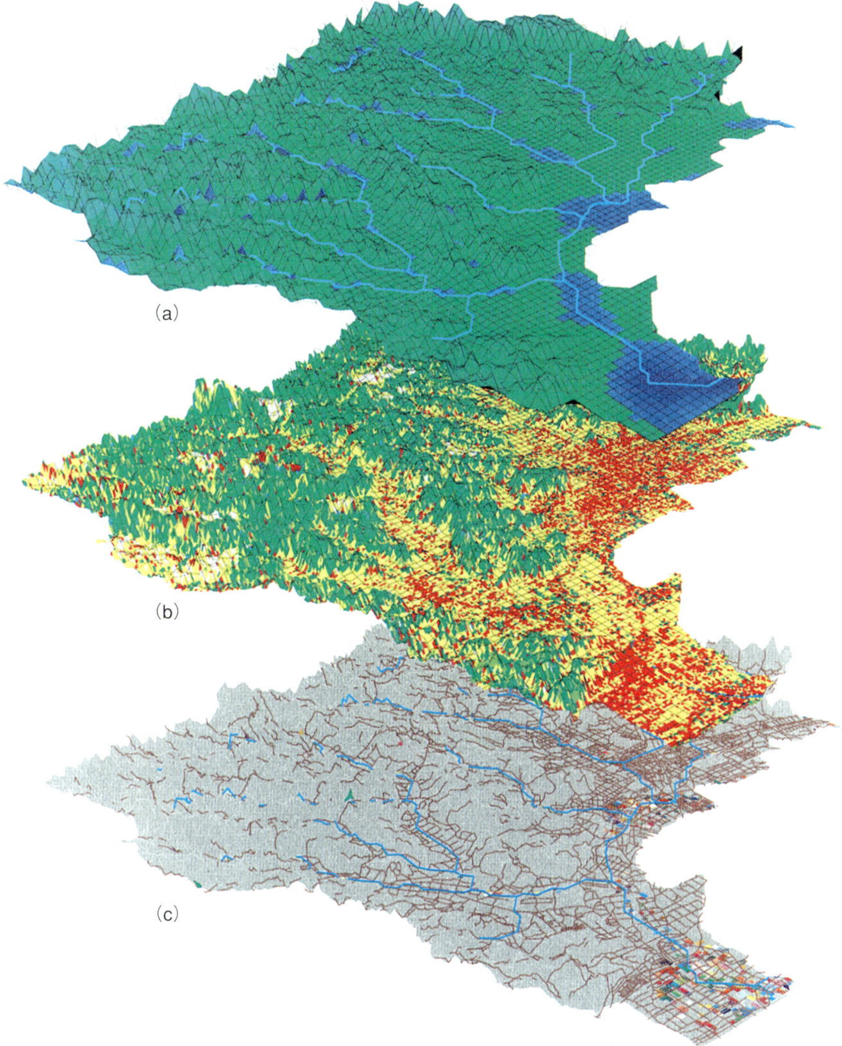

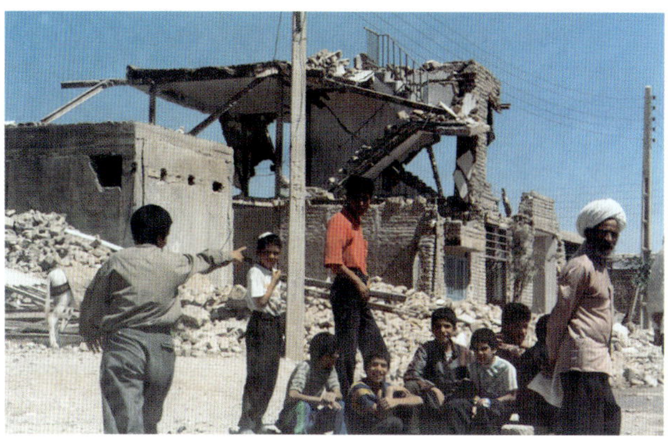

Site ivestigation of damaged area by natural hazards

Although it is impossible to reduce the number of hazards which are natural phenomena, International Center for Disaster-Mitigation Engineering (INCEDE) believes that the level of a disaster, that is the total effects of damage due to a hazard, can be reduced. INCEDE staff visit the disaster-affected areas to investigate and obtain first-hand information and data. This data is compiled and stored in a disaster database. Using the INCEDE network, the data is distributed to members. The photograph, taken at Gayen in Northeast Iran, shows the damage to buildings caused by the Quyen earthquake of May 1997.

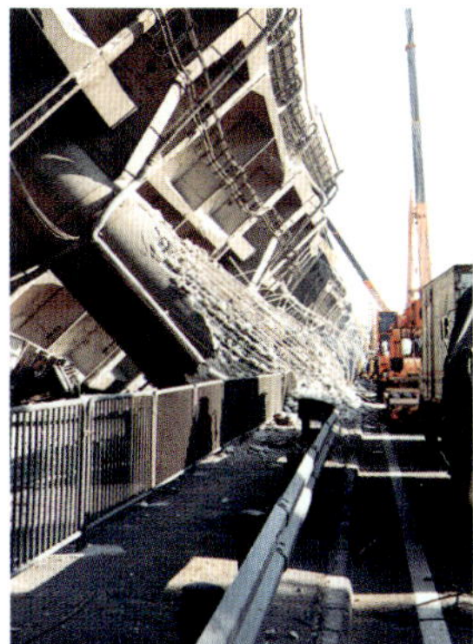

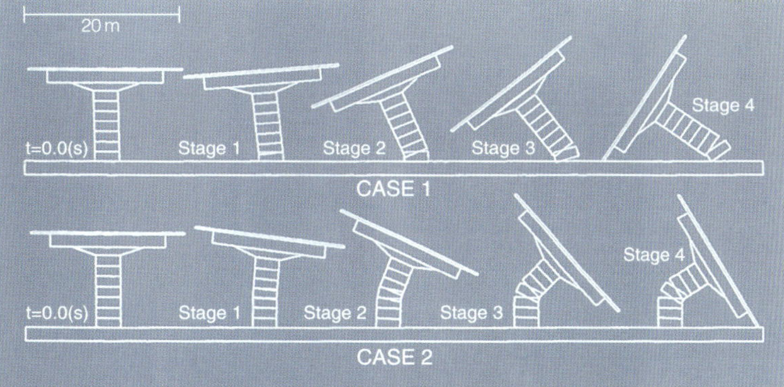

Simulation of collapse process of elevated expressway bridges due to the 1995 Hyogoken-Nanbu Earthquake

To mitigate casualties due to earthquakes, it is important to study the mechanism of the collapse of structures during earthquakes. Using a newly developed model, the collapse mechanism of buildings and infrastructure during the 1995 Hyogo ken-Nanbu Earthquake has been studied through the simulation of various modes of collapse process of structures, especially that of elevated expressway bridges as reported after the quake. The new model is applicable to both a composite and continuous medium, and a fully discrete one. Although the phenomena treated in this study were difficult to simulate by conventional methods such as the finite element method, the numerical results obtained agree well with the actual earthquake damage.

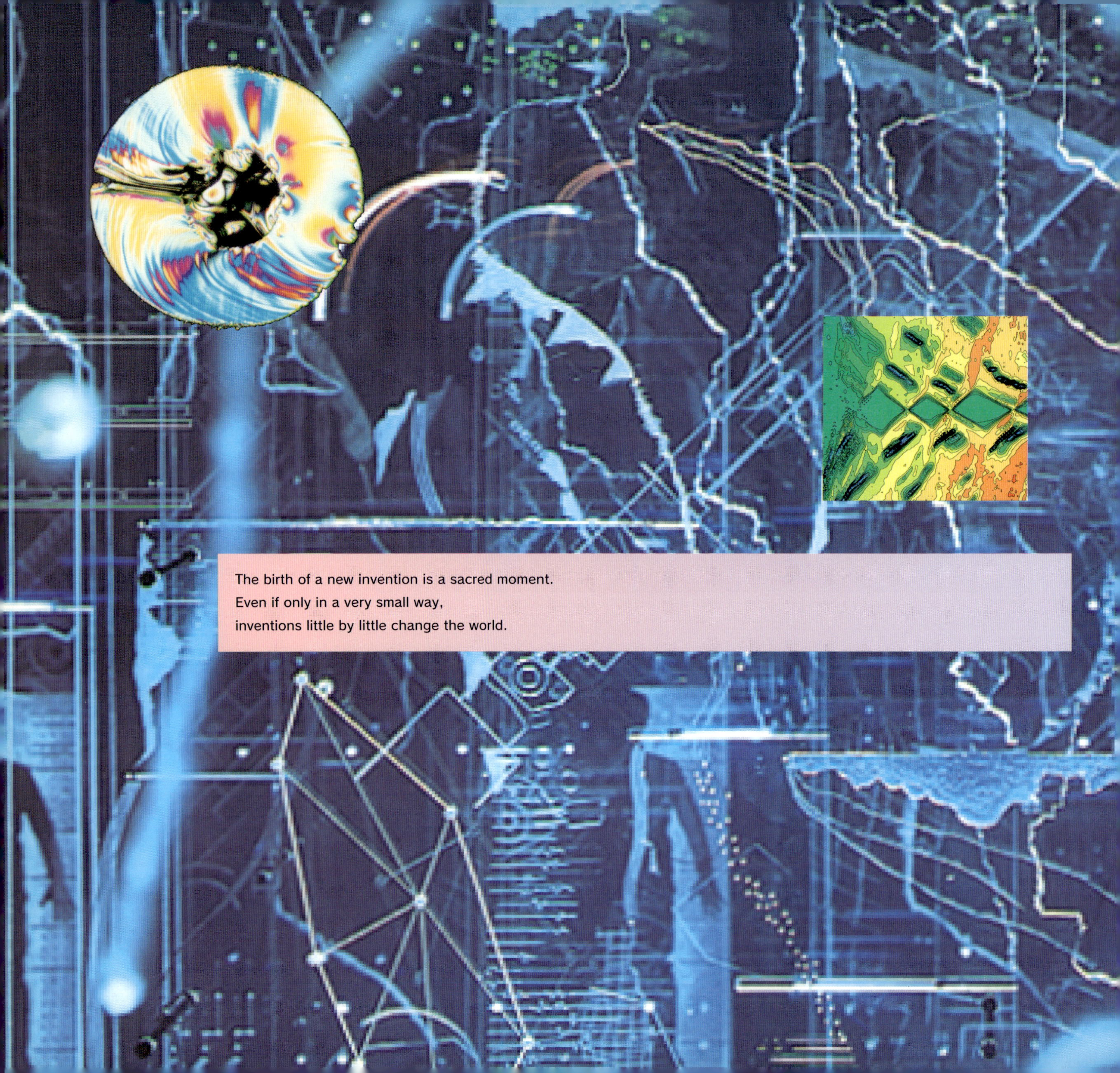
The birth of a new invention is a sacred moment.
Even if only in a very small way,
inventions little by little change the world.

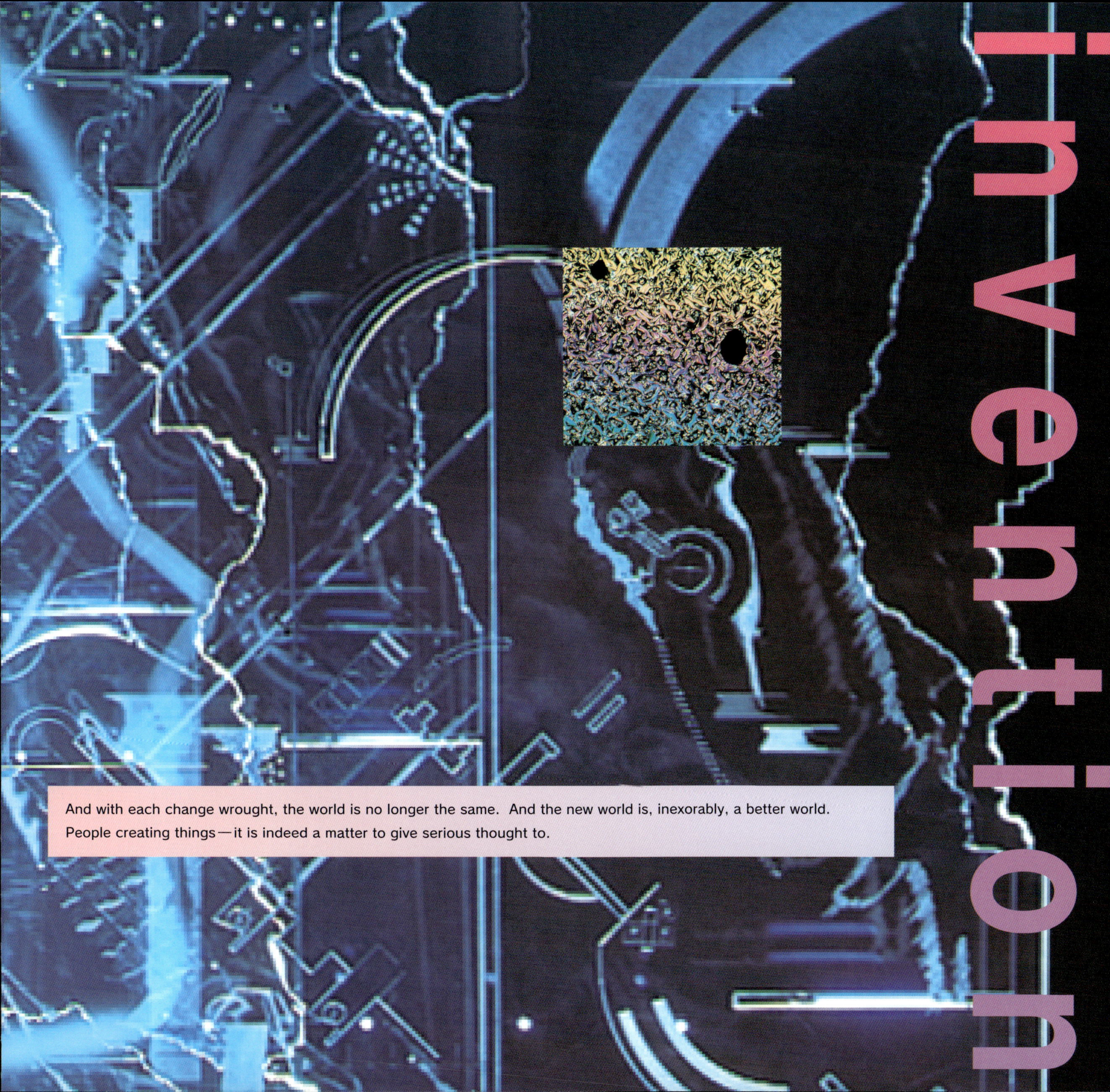

invention

And with each change wrought, the world is no longer the same. And the new world is, inexorably, a better world.
People creating things—it is indeed a matter to give serious thought to.

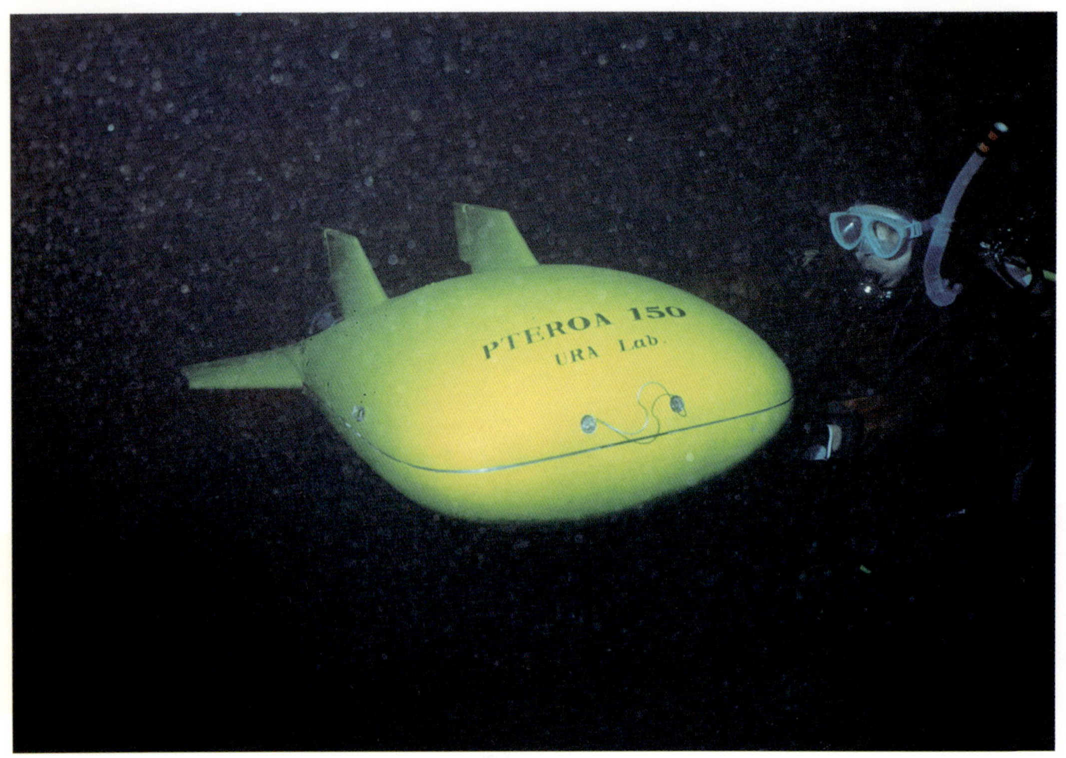

Underwater robot "PTEROA150"

Autonomous underwater robots are under development based on new technologies which can dive as "Atom Boys" perfectly free from restriction from operators on the surface ship. The "PTEROA 150", constructed in 1988 as the first Japanese prototype robot, is a compact vehicle 220 kg in weight, which glides down to the bottom and cruises above the bed based on range data from acoustic ranging sensors.

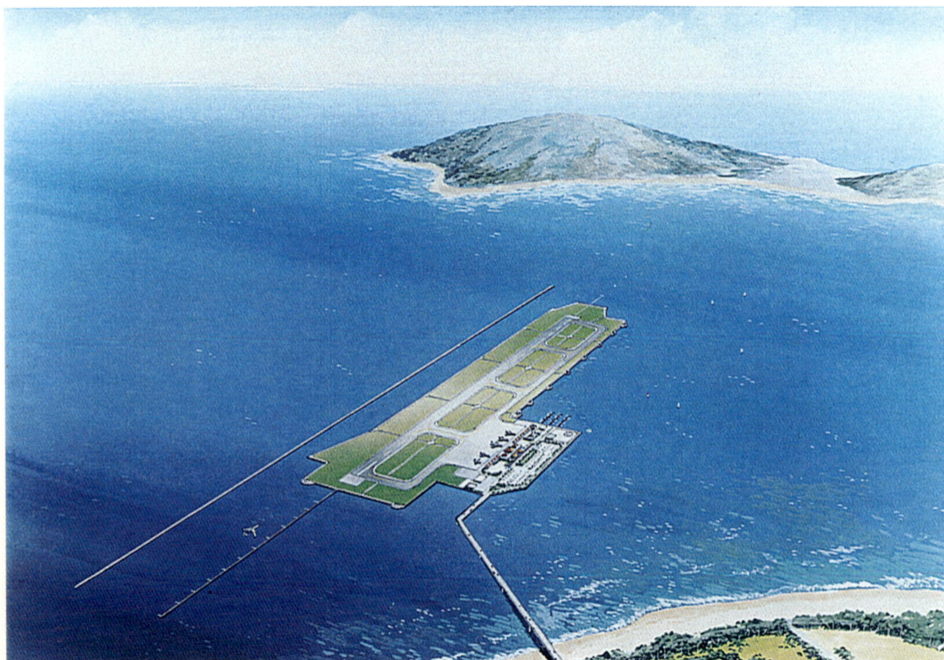

Artist's image of a medium size floating airport

The most expected application of Mega-Float is as a floating airport which is friendly to the ocean environment, strong against earthquakes, and with easy mobility and removal. Its length is 2 to 5 km, its breadth 500 to 1,000 m, and draught up to 3 m. It is now feasible to design a floating airport which satisfies safety criteria for strength and position-keeping even in typhoons, and has the safety of an automatic landing system in a high sea state. (figure by Courtesy of Mega-Float Technical Research Association)

The sea is a treasure house of resources. The resources increase if the sea can be used more, by searching out the resources using underwater robots, or by constructing huge floating facilities. We need to consider how to make maximum usage of the sea, because Japan is surrounded by sea.

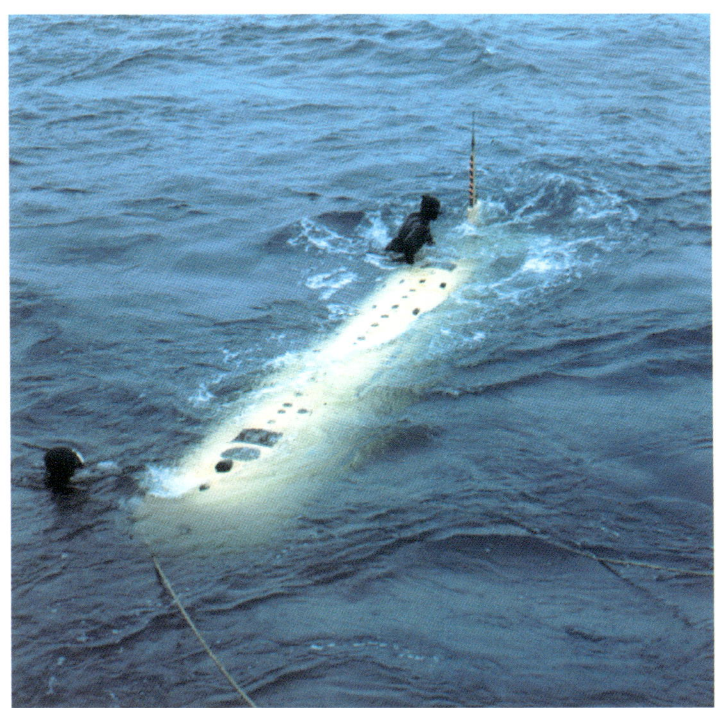

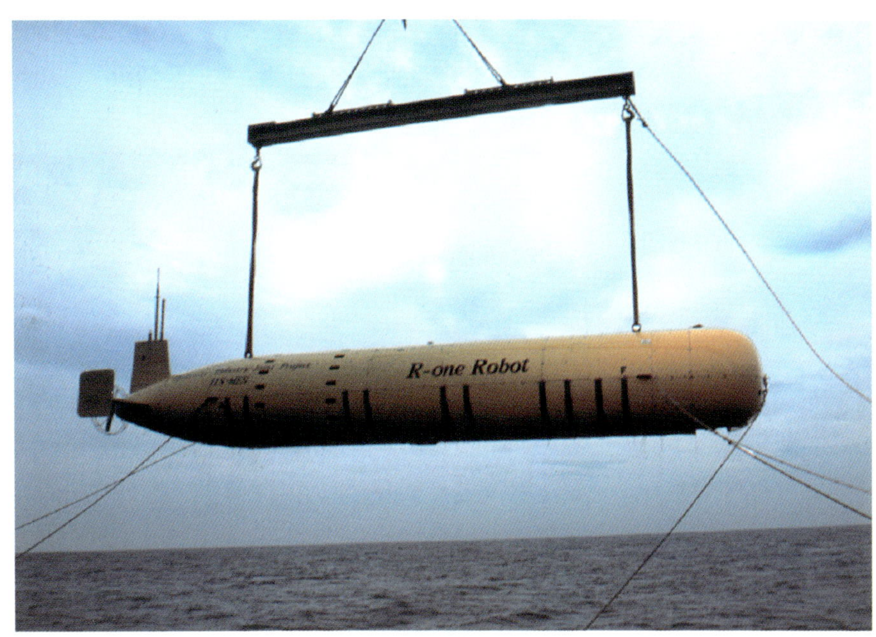

R-one robot

Some robots should cruise for a long range to cover wide area of the oceans. The "R-one Robot", which is equipped with a closed cycle diesel engine system as its energy source, is 4 tons in weight and 8 meters in length, succeeded in cruising for 70 km in 12 hours on June 16th 1998, and demonstrated its capability as an underwater platform.

Mega-Float elastic model test in directional waves

Mega-Float (Very Large Floating Structure) behaves as a membrane in directional ocean waves due to its low rigidity. In order to confirm the strength safety, or the safety function of an automatic landing system for an airport under wave conditions, a corresponding elastic model test in directional waves is required.

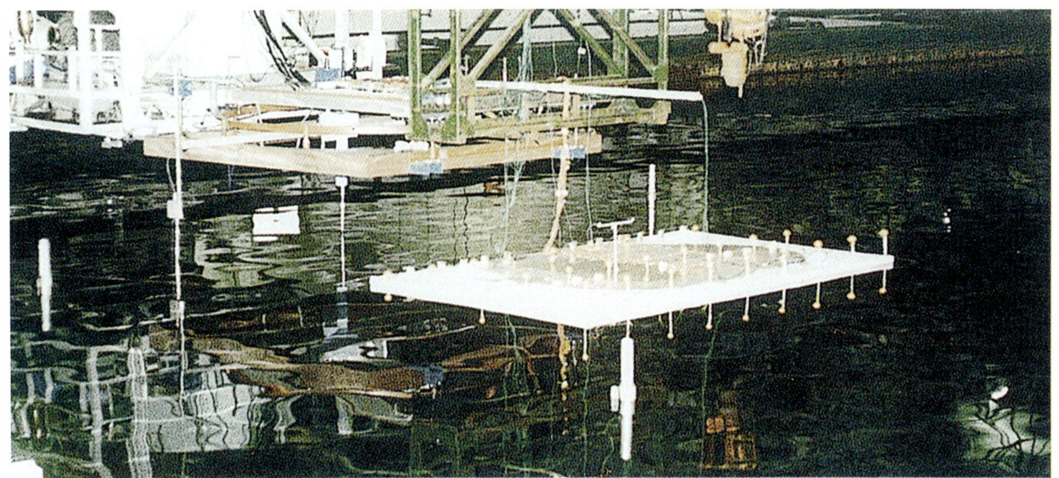

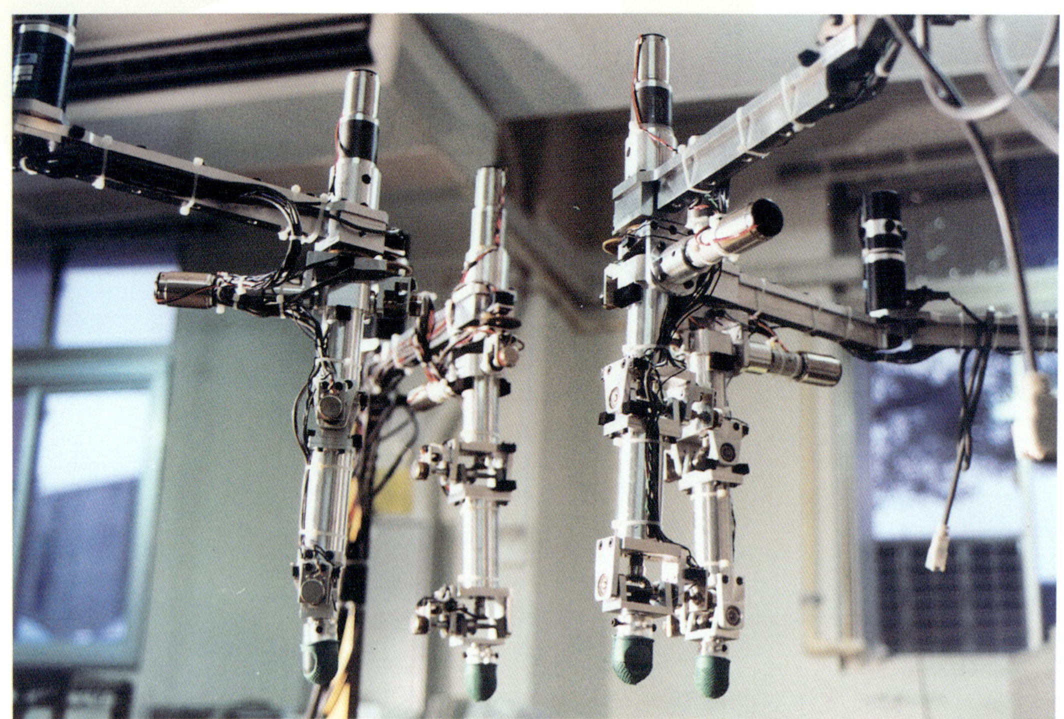

Dexterous Robot Hand

A Dexterous Robot Hand has been developed to do research on human-like skill in robotics. This hand is composed of 4 fingers, each of which has 6-degrees of freedom and a 6-axis force sensor. This hand is controlled at a 1 msec sampling period in order to achieve dexterous manipulation such as grasping.

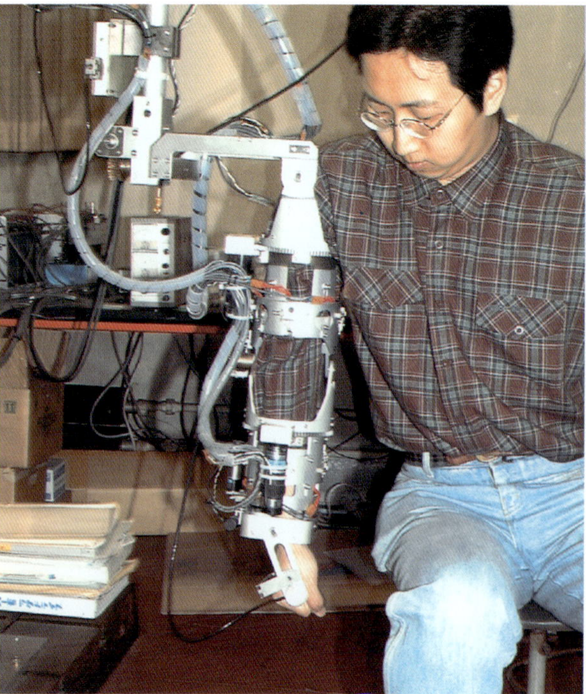

Sensor Arm

The Sensor Arm is an arm-type 7-degree of freedom haptic interface, and can make force feedback at each joint of the human arm. This arm can be utilized as an interface for interactive communication with the virtual environment and as a master manipulator of a tele-operation system.

Sensor Glove II

The Sensor Glove II is a glove-shaped 20-degree of freedom haptic interface, which can feed back realistic force through actuators to each joint of the human hand handling virtual objects. This glove will enable us to feel as if we were touching objects in virtual space.

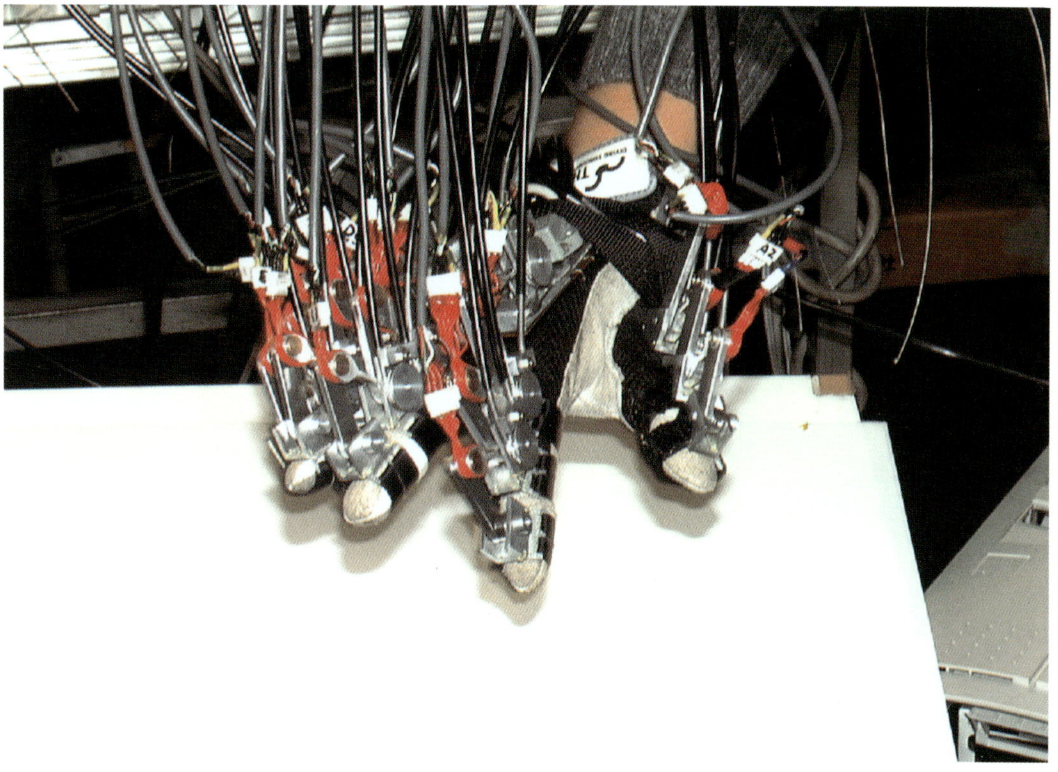

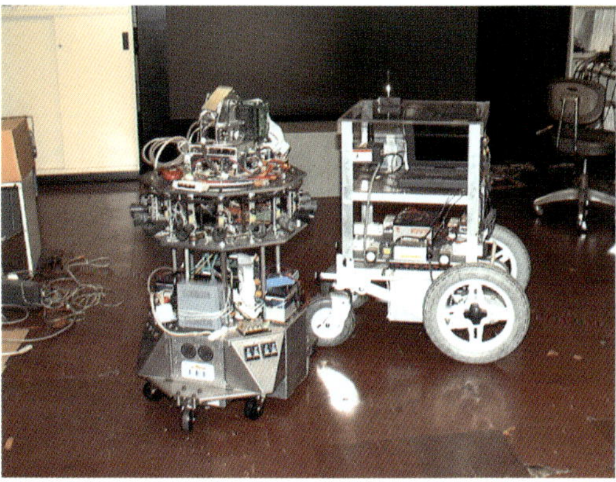

Mobile Robot

A Mobile Robot has been developed to conduct research on the coexistence of humans and robots. This robot can move omnidirectionally by using two motors per each driving wheel. This robot knows its own position and can recognize obstacles and humans by cooperating with its surrounding environment including sensors such as cameras.

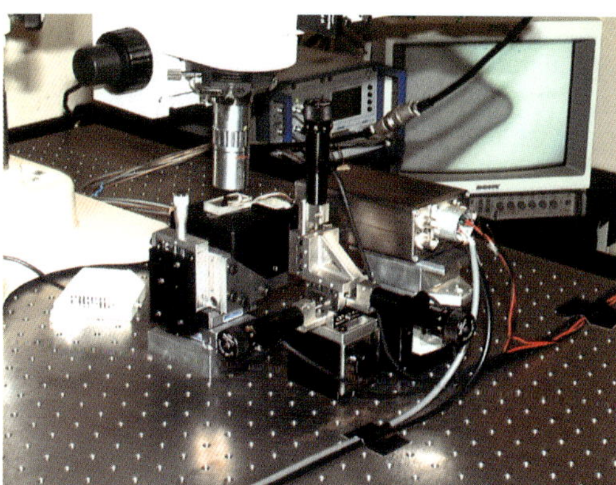

AFM

These pieces of equipment are composed of an antivibration table, an optical microscope and an Atomic Force Microscope (AFM). AFM was originally developed to image surfaces with atomic resolution, and has recently been used to modify surfaces at the nanometer scale. This has even achieved the manipulation and positioning of micro-scale particles on a surface.

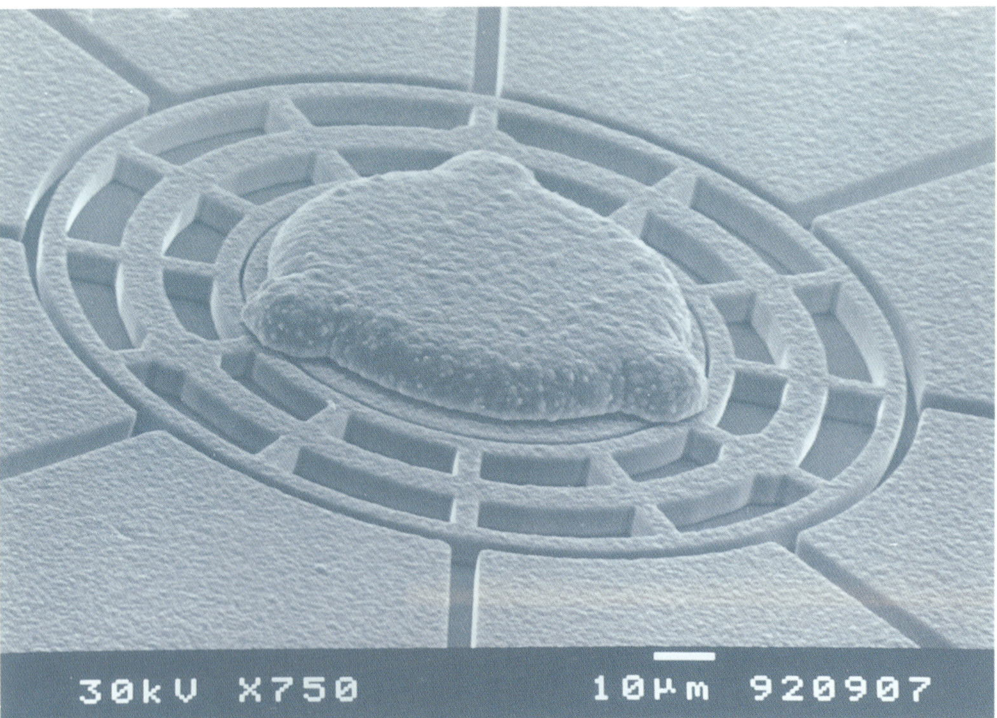

(a)

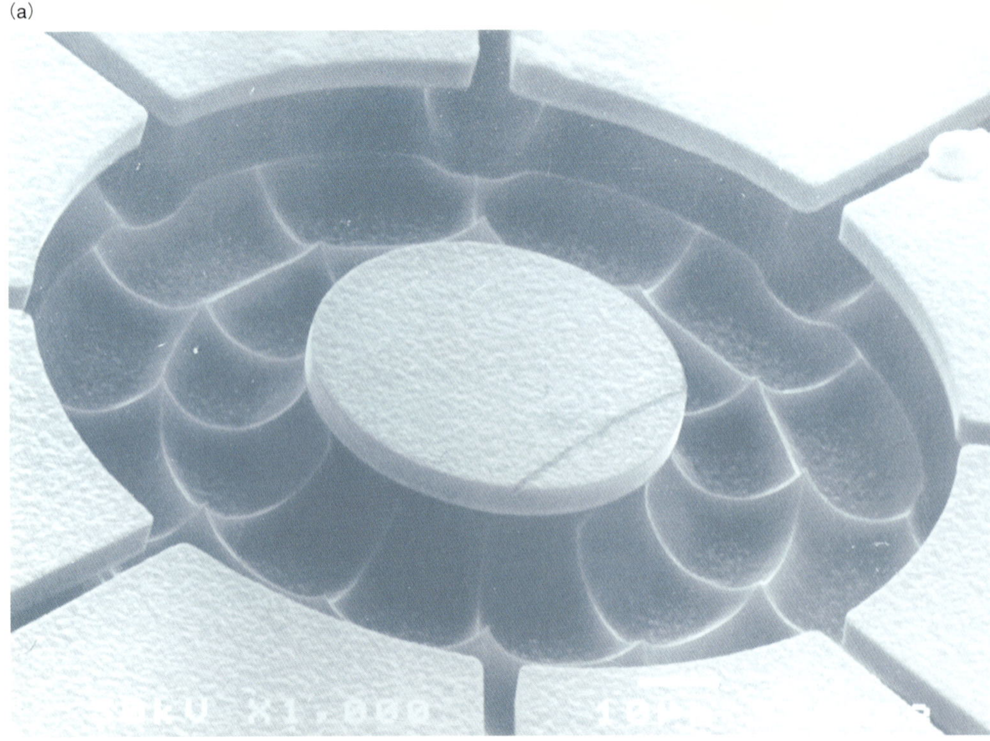

(b)

Micro motor driven by electrostatic force

Micro motors can be as small as a human hair (diameter 100 μm, thickness 7 μm). The rotor inside is attracted to the stators outside step by step to rotate around the axis. Maximum speed is ten thousand revolutions a minute. The structure was made by electroplating of nickel into a mold, formed by photolithography. The bottom picture shows the base substrate after the rotor has been removed, showing how the rotor was released by plasma etching of underlying silicon.

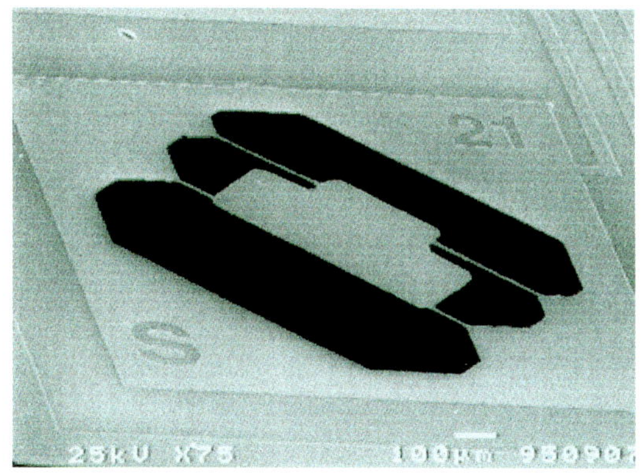

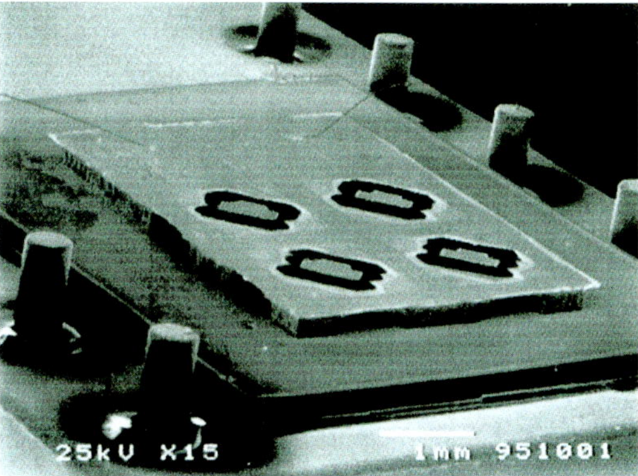

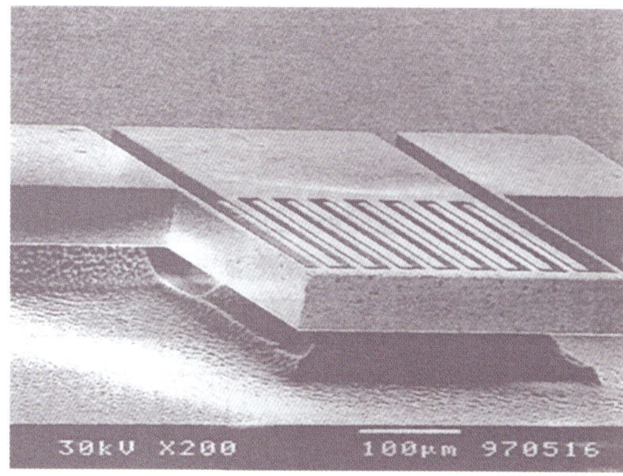

Silicon torsion mirrors for light communications

A large number of optical fibers of low insertion loss and high switching contrast are required for optical fiber networks and local area networks for computers. Micromachining technology enables us to make micro mirrors (0.4 mm) for insertion into the light beam emitted from an optical fiber, to change the optical pass by reflecting the beams. We have demonstrated good optical switching performance.

Micro actuator for ultrahigh density disk storage system

The trend of hard-disk technology toward small size and high density is so rapid that the data density is increasing by 60% a year. Micro actuators are expected to control the pick-up head position precisely and quickly for reading / writing data bits at high accuracy. The figure shows an electrostatic actuator of 50 microns high and minimum 2.5 microns wide. We demonstrated that the device has the performance to meet the requirements of hard disk technology.

Poly-Si 3-D micro structures

By depositing a film of 1 to 2 microns in thickness onto a silicon substrate and patterning it by micro technique, one can make microscale structures, as if cutting out planar patterns from thick paper. To make them into 3-D structures, people usually fold the thin patterns. On the other hand, we can use Joule heat with an electrical current up to 600 to 700 degrees C; the micro parts are softened by the heat and one can fold it up easily. The figure shows an example of a micro 3-D structure formed after the reshaping technique of Joule heat.

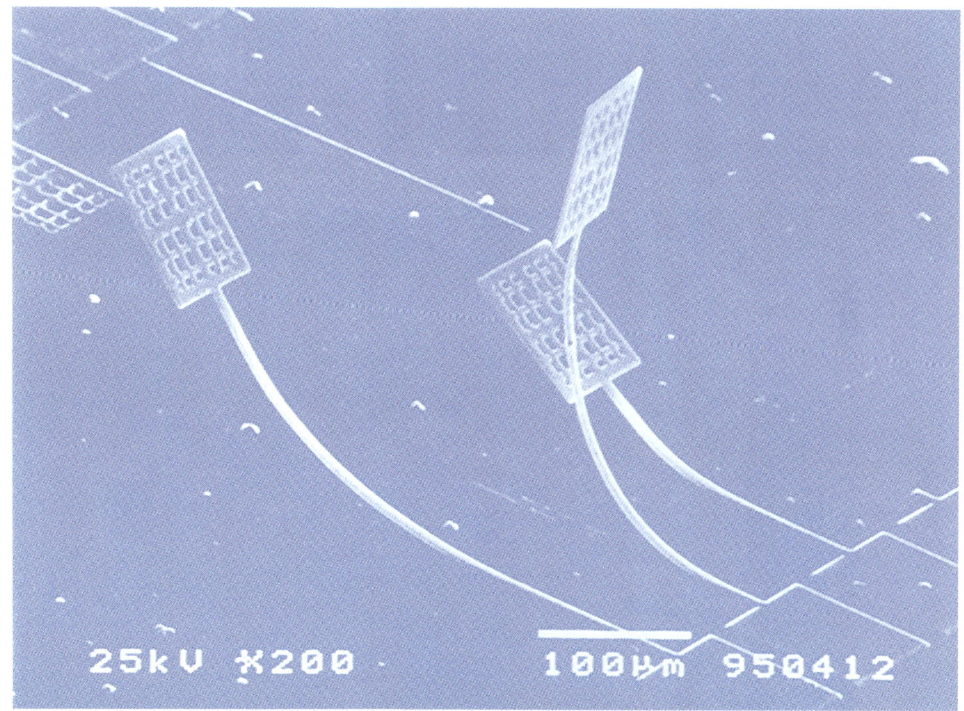

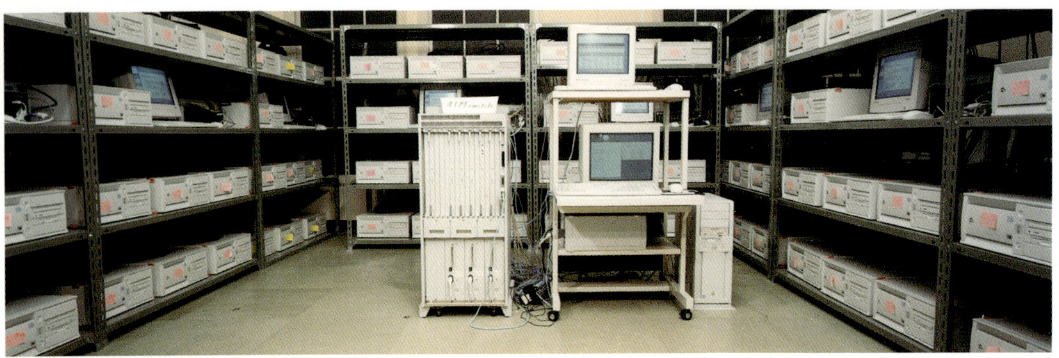

100-node PC cluster system

The cost of personal computers is decreasing significantly, so we may be able to build a super-computer by connecting large number of PC's. NEDO-100 is a 100 node PC cluster system, where nodes are linked through an ATM switch. Parallel data warehousing and parallel data mining were implemented on it, which shows much higher performance than expensive server machines.

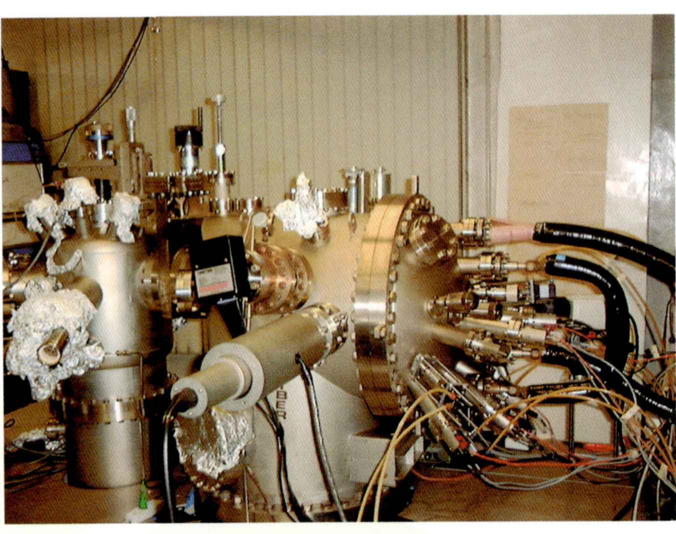

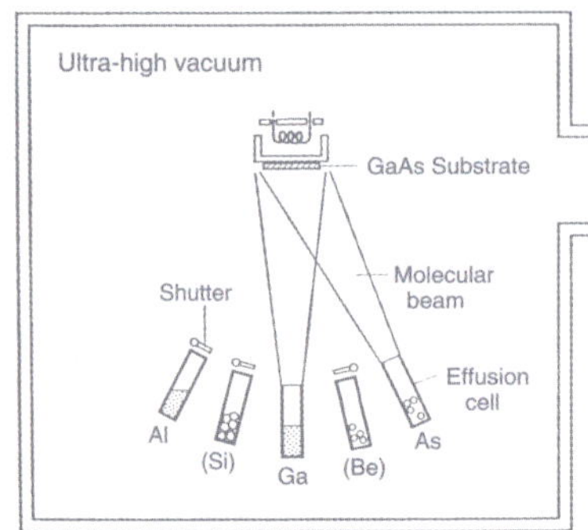

Molecular beam epitaxy and semiconductor nano-structures

Molecular beams can be generated in an ultra-high vacuum chamber by heating a set of source materials in crucibles. After arriving at an appropriate crystalline substrate, these molecules react and result in layer-by-layer growth of semiconductor films. In I.I.S. we initiated research on molecular beam epitaxy in 1979, and since then, we have developed a variety of original hetero-structures. The cross-sectional TEM image shows a single AlAs molecular layer (0.3 nm) embedded in GaAs. These structures play crucial roles in advanced electronic devices used especially for communication systems.

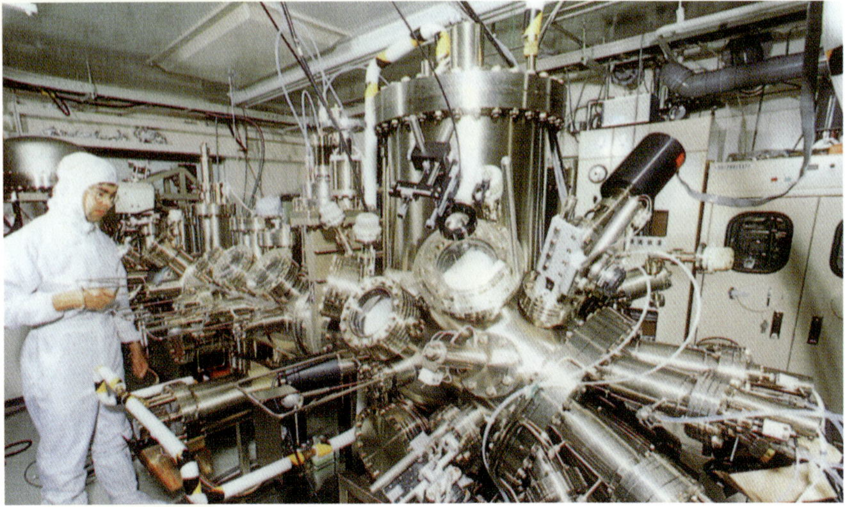

Atomic level characterization and control of semiconductor heterojunctions

When ultrathin semiconductor films of the order of 10 nm are stacked, the motion of confined electrons are quantized. Such quantum heterostructures exhibit unique properties and are expected to play important roles in future ultrafast optoelectronic devices. The photo shows an ultra high vacuum system in which stacks of ultrathin semiconductor materials can be grown with atomic resolution (molecular beam epitaxy) and their electronic structures can be studied in situ by X-ray photo-emission (photoelectron spectroscopy).

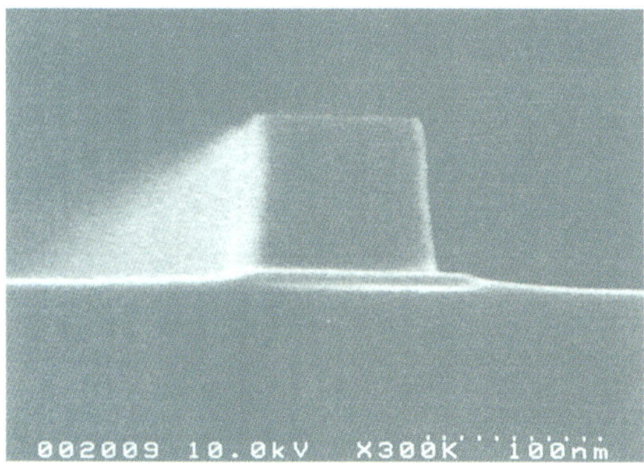

Sub-0.1 µm SOI VLSI device

Thin film SOI MOSFETs are promising for very low power VLSI devices. Sub-0.1 µm SOI devices were successfully fabricated using electron beam lithography. The floating body effects caused by the impact ionization current were intensively investigated below 1 V.

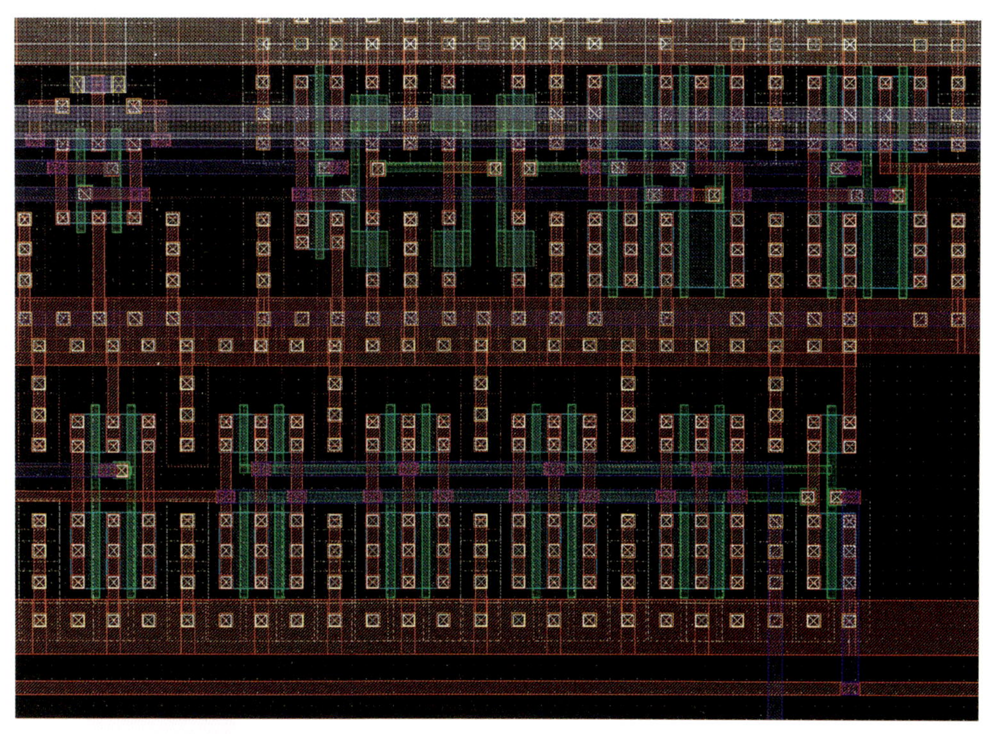

Super Cut-off CMOS Scheme

Recently the power consumption of CMOS VLSI's is increasing rapidly, and heat and battery life problems are becoming increasingly eminent. In order to make a breakthrough, it is effective to decrease the supply voltage down to sub 1 V because the power depends quadratically on the supply voltage. MOS transistors, however, cannot be turned on and CMOS (Complimentaly Metal Oxide Semiconductor) circuits cannot work properly if the supply voltage is less than 0.6 V, since the turn-on voltage of MOS transistors is about 0.6 V. The SCCMOS scheme is proposed and demonstrated to provide high speed CMOS VLSI (Very Large Scale Integration) even when the supply voltage is less than 0.6 V.

Artificial micro ear by silicon micromachining

The basilar membrane in an inner ear has a function of real time frequency analysis for auditory systems. We have developed an artificial basilar membrane by silicon micromachining. Silicon cantilevers of different lengths are arrayed and they respond to the input mechanical vibration through their resonant frequencies.

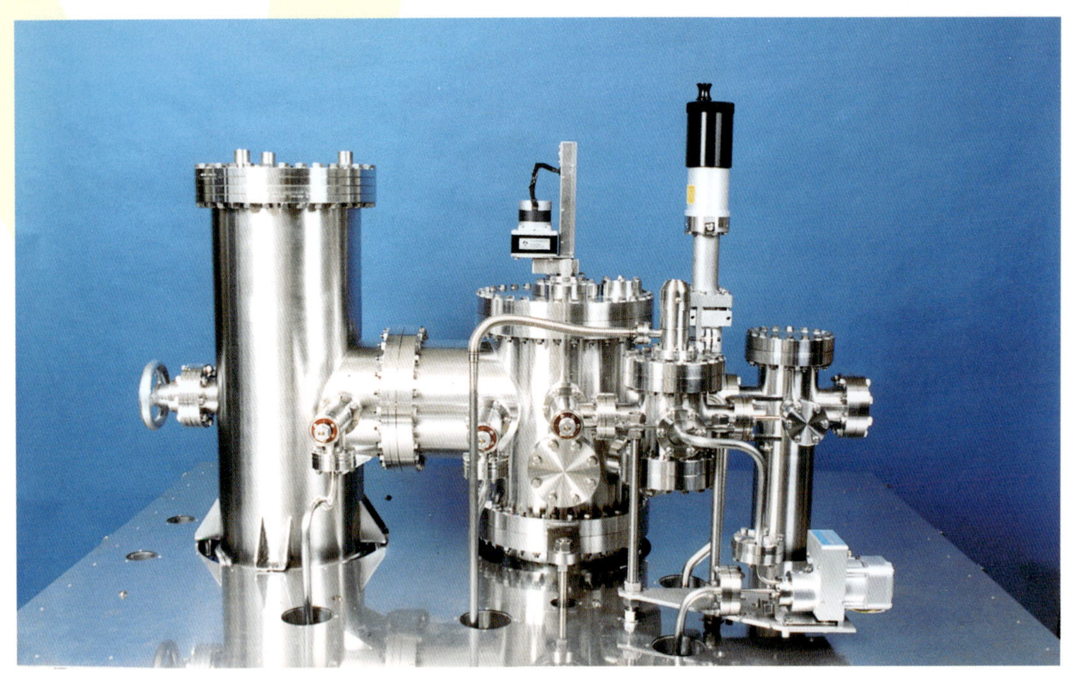

Diagnosis of extremely-high vacuum

Recent advances in individual atom manipulation on solid surfaces requires an ultimate contamination-free environment. Extremely high vacuum has become an important condition in realizing such an environment. The apparatus shown in the photo was developed for the accurate measurement of outgassing rates and pumping speeds in a vacuum vessel at pressures as low as 10^{-10} Pa.

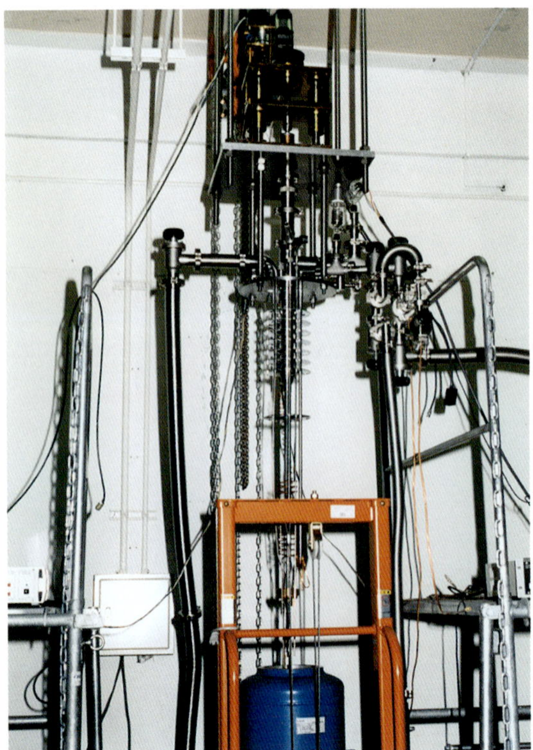

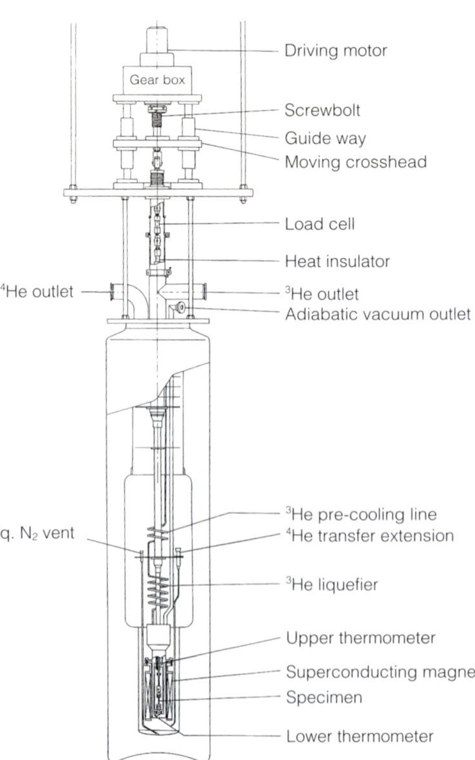

Low temperature mechanical testing device

The plastic deformation of materials occurs by the motion of dislocation. The picture shows a device for the investigation of the quantum effect on dislocation motion in metals and ionic crystals at temperatures close to the absolute zero. A sample in a cryostat at the bottom is cooled down to 0.5 K by liquid ^{3}He. A tensile-test apparatus at the top deforms the sample very slowly.

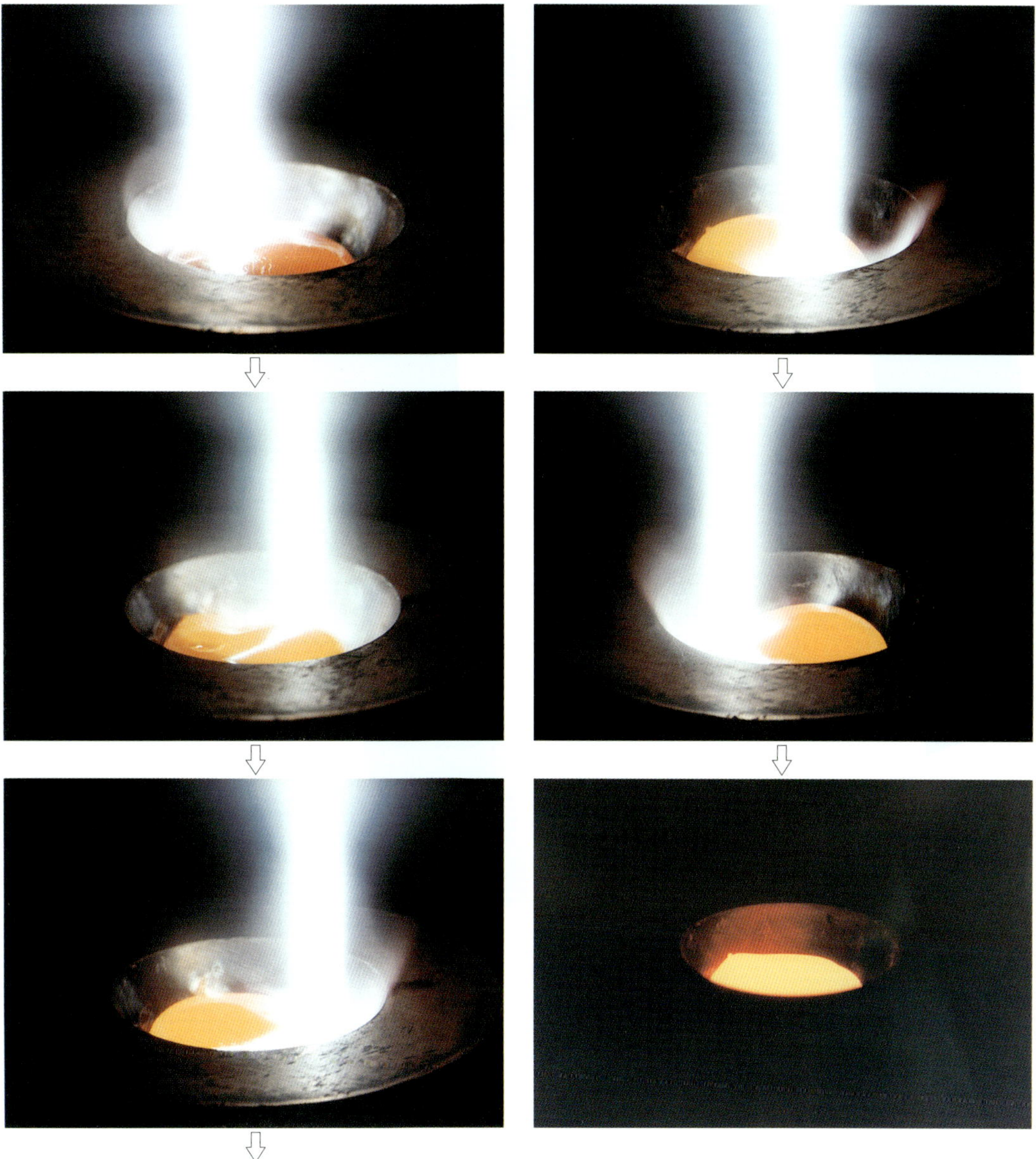

Plasma arc remelting of refractory and less noble metals and their alloy

As a heat source, plasma arc is used for various industrial processes for refining and remelting. This apparatus has a transfer type torch with a rotational device. To maximize the use of heat and to control the momentum of plasma gas, the radius and rate of rotation can be varied by the device during melting. This figure shows the rotating plasma arc and molten titanium in a water-cooled copper crucible.

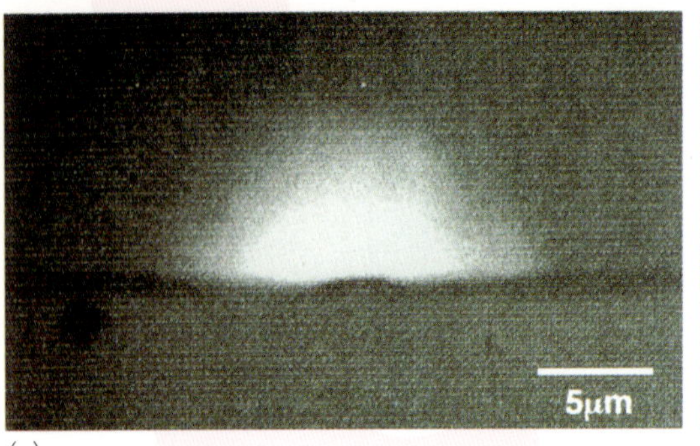

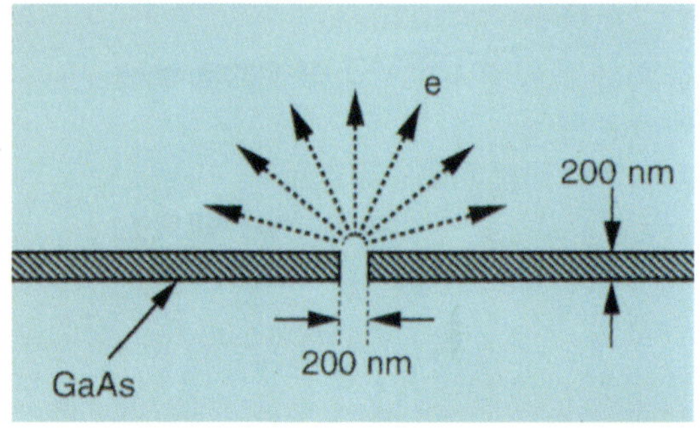

Visualization of electron flow in ultra small semiconductor point contact

In semiconductors such as GaAs, electrons with excess energy radiate photons (luminescence). By imaging this luminescence with a microscope, the state inside the device can be detected. This method is applied to a 200 nm wide point contact structure where a pair of wedge-shaped grooves are introduced into a conducting film of InGaAs to investigate the radal electron flow from the constriction. As the electron flow influences (weakens) luminescence, the electron flow is successfully visualized. By extending this technique, time-resolved movements of an electron packet can also be observed.

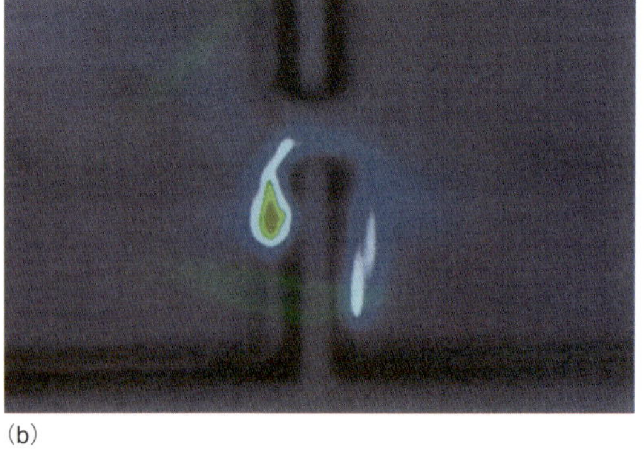

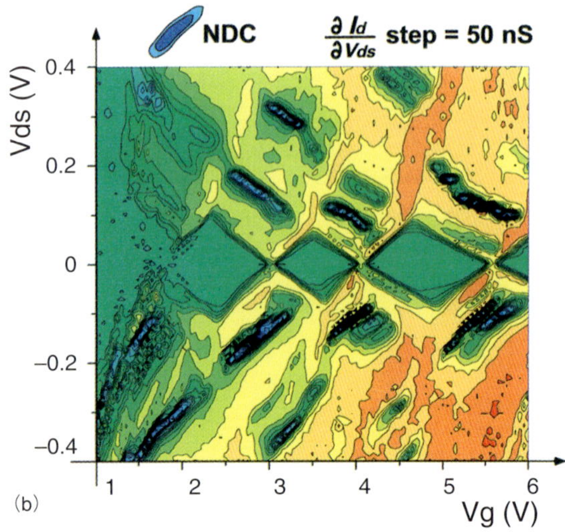

Blue nitride-semiconductor surface emitting lasers →

Blue surface emitting lasers attract increasing interest since it is expected that two-dimensional arrays of blue laser diodes should drastically reduce the read-out time in optical memories. The figure shows schematically the structure of the blue surface emitting laser grown by MOCVD and its optical properties. The measurement was performed at 77 K under optical excitation. Lasing emission was confirmed by observing that the spectral linewidth was as sharp as 0.1 nm.

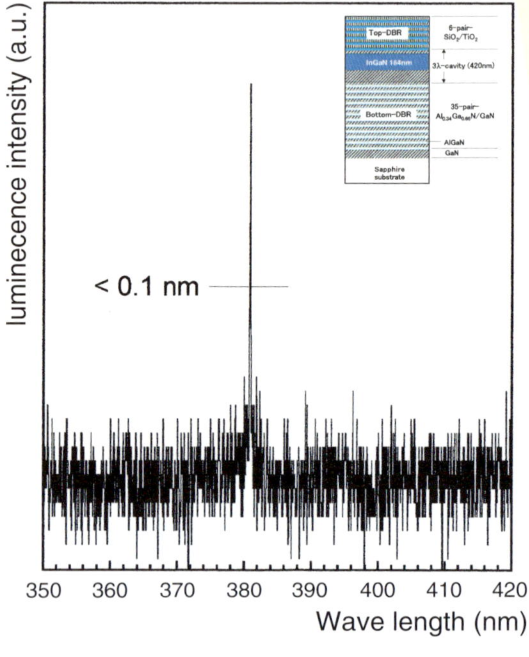

← Silicon single electron transistor operating at room temperature

A silicon single electron transistor operating at room temperature were successfully fabricated using VLSI-compatible process. The coulomb blockade oscillations were clearly observed (fig. (a)). The quantum effects in such a small device were also intensively studied (fig. (b)).

Single dot spectroscopy by using nano-probing techniques

We can investigate single dot spectroscopy by using nano-probing techniques, e.g. Near-field Scanning Optical Microscope (NSOM) and Scanning Tunneling Microsope (STM). The figures show the principle of the NSOM and spatial evolution of the photo-luminescence spectra in different spin states of InGaAs quantum dots (the pairs of luminescence lines show Zeeman splitting in the magnetic field).

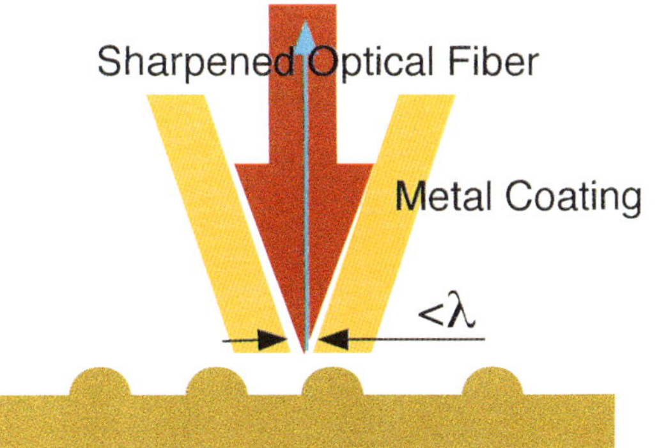

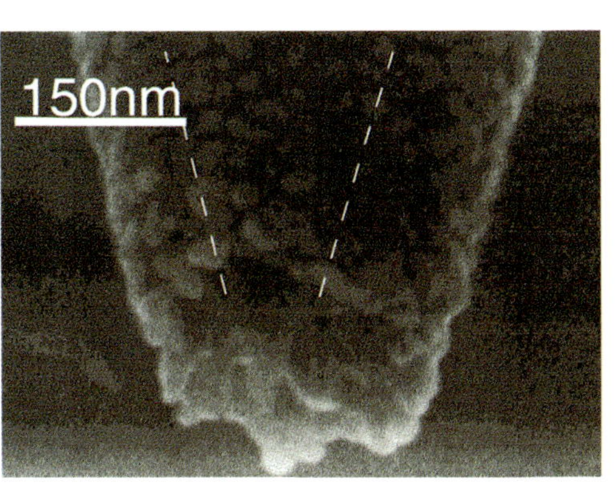

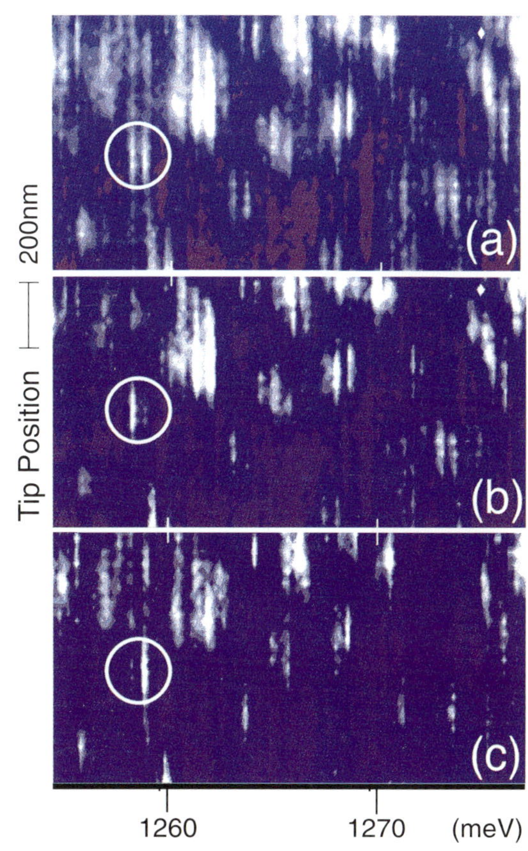

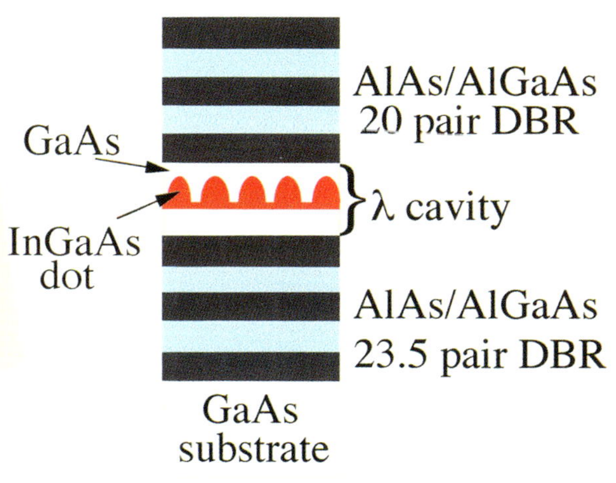

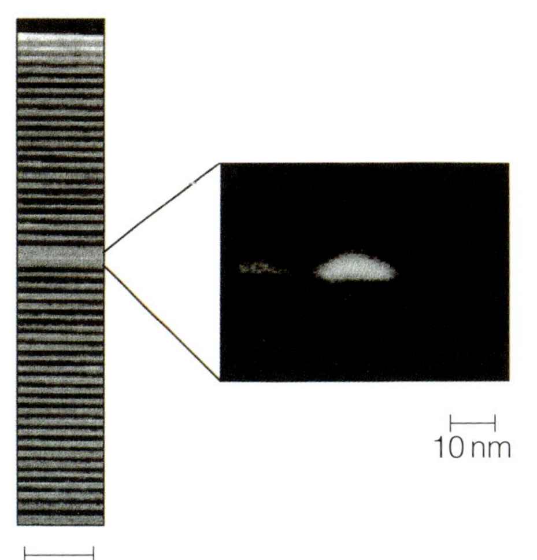

Microcavity quantum dot lasers

The control of both electron and photon modes in confined structures should play an important role in the optical devices for future communication systems. We successfully fabricated a vertical microcavity quantum dot laser with lasing oscillation at 77 K. The InGaAs quantum dots were grown by the Stranski-Krastnanow growth mode with the MOCVD. The lasing oscillation at the first sub-band of quantum dots by tuning the resonant wavelength of the microcavity to the corresponding photon energy.

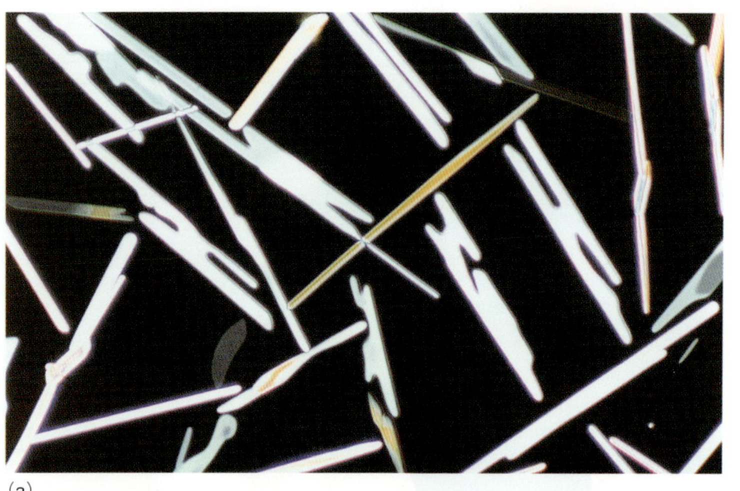

(a)

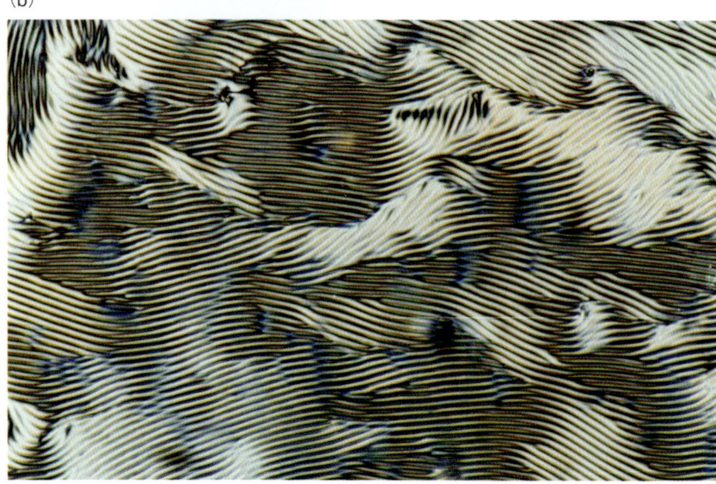

(b)

(c)

Supramolecular liquid crystals

Liquid crystal is a unique organic molecular system, which is now widely used for advanced materials such as display devices. For further applications for high-tech and bio-technologies, supramolecular liquid crystals have been designed and built through self-assembly of a variety of organic molecules. The pictures show polarizing microscope images of these liquid crystals with molecular self-organized structures.

Molecular photonics switch

Molecular devices can be envisaged as minuscule photo/electronic devices, which are constituted from molecule-based components. Upon light excitation of a metal complex containing ruthenium (shown as a green circle) and osmium (red circle) ions, energy transfers from the former to the latter site from where the output light-emission comes out. This complex serves as a molecular switch, since the energy transfer process can be switched on/off by injecting/ejecting an electron through an external source. The separation between the ruthenium and osmium centers is in the order of one nano-meter.

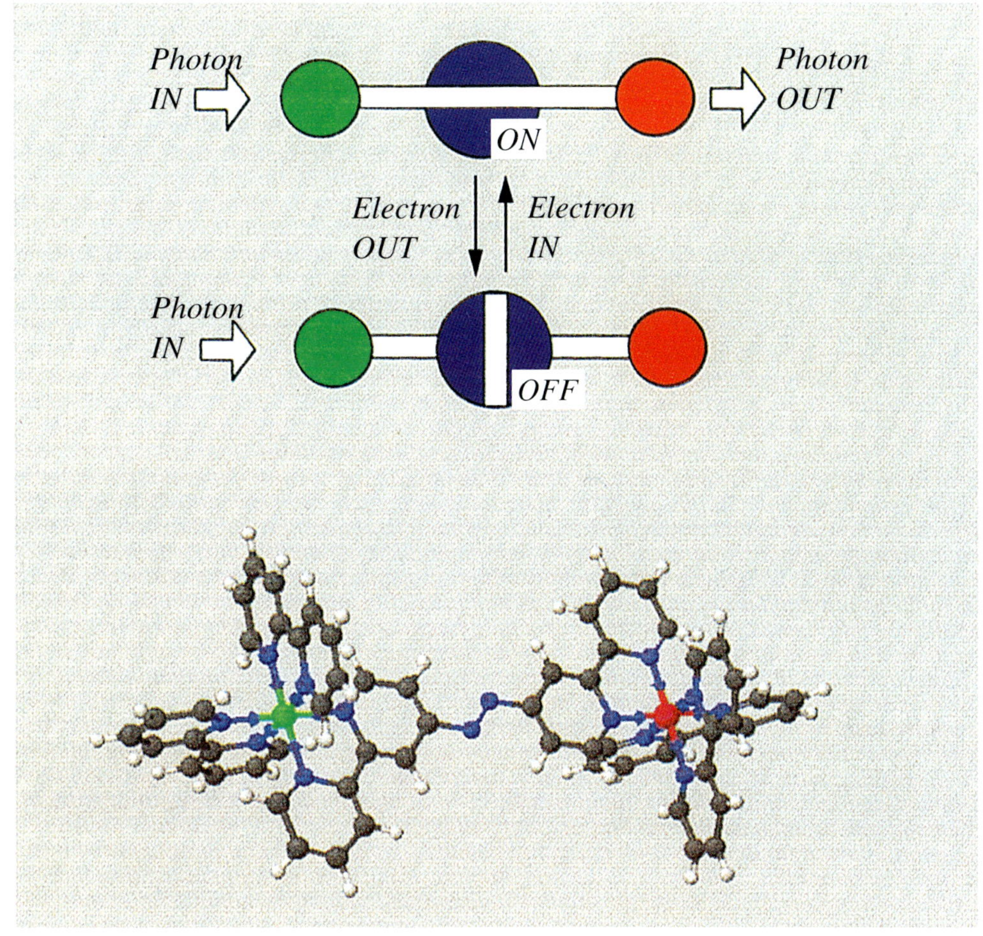

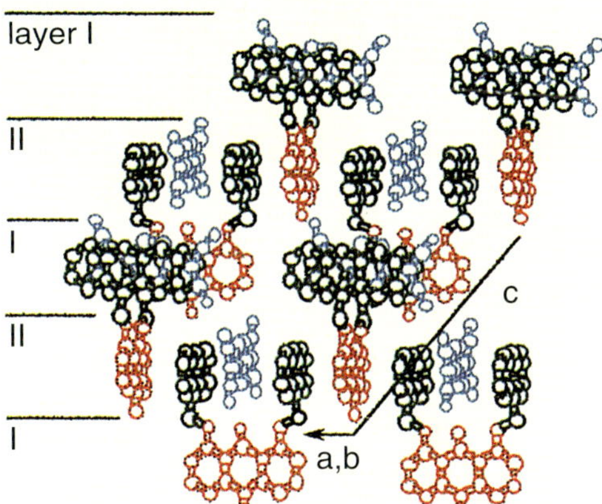

Organic Charge-transfer superstructure

As a part of our research program to design photo/electro-active nano-architecture, an organic charge transfer superstructure was self-assembled by using the donor-acceptor interaction. The figure shows a superlattice-like crystal structure composed of alternating 0.63 nm-thick differently-oriented layers which are arrays of columns made up from stacked donors (black) and acceptors (red and blue).

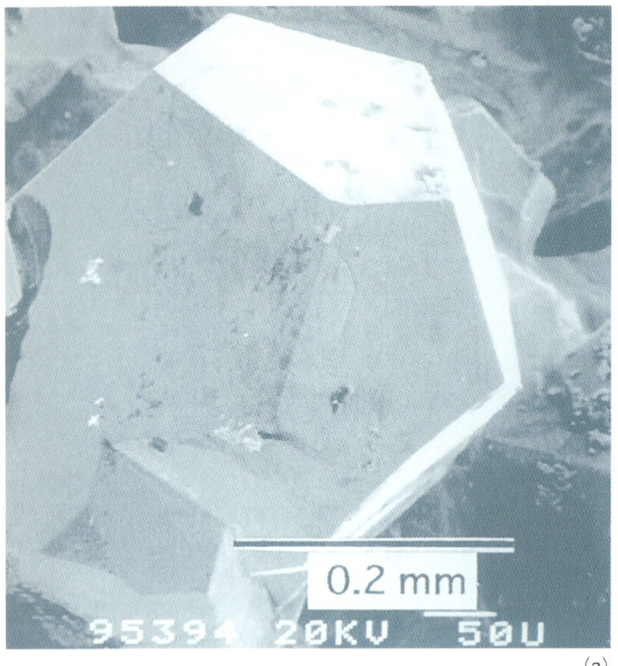

(a)

(b)

Single quasicrystal in Al-Cu-Ru alloy

Crystal means a periodic arrangement of atoms. Quasicrystals have also long range order but have aperiodic structures. A single quasicrystal of Al-Cu-Ru has a regular dodecahedral-like shape (fig. (a)) and shows a flower like an X-ray Laue pattern, which reflects the symmetry of the atomic arrangement (fig. (b)). Both of them show a five-fold rotational symmetry, which cannot be allowed in any crystals.

Thin film material for saving-energy smart windows

VO_2 shows a semiconductor-to-metal transition at $T_c=67\,°C$ with a dramatic decrease in the transmittance of near infrared rays. Thus thin film is applicable for smart windows. We have developed a coating technique of VO_2 film doped with tungsten or molybdenum to lower the Tc utilizing our original soft chemical method, which is needed from a practical point of view.

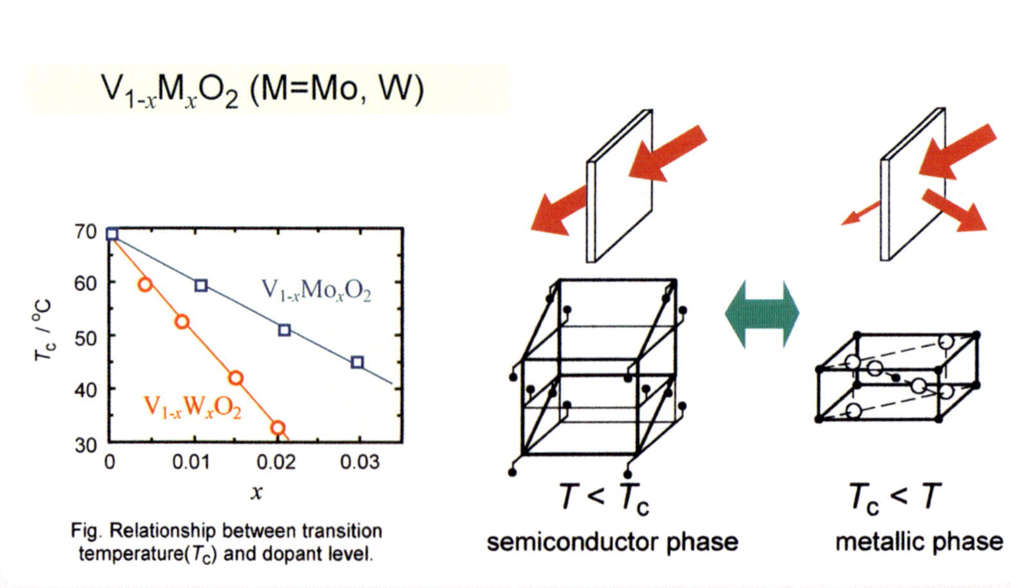

Fig. Relationship between transition temperature(T_c) and dopant level.

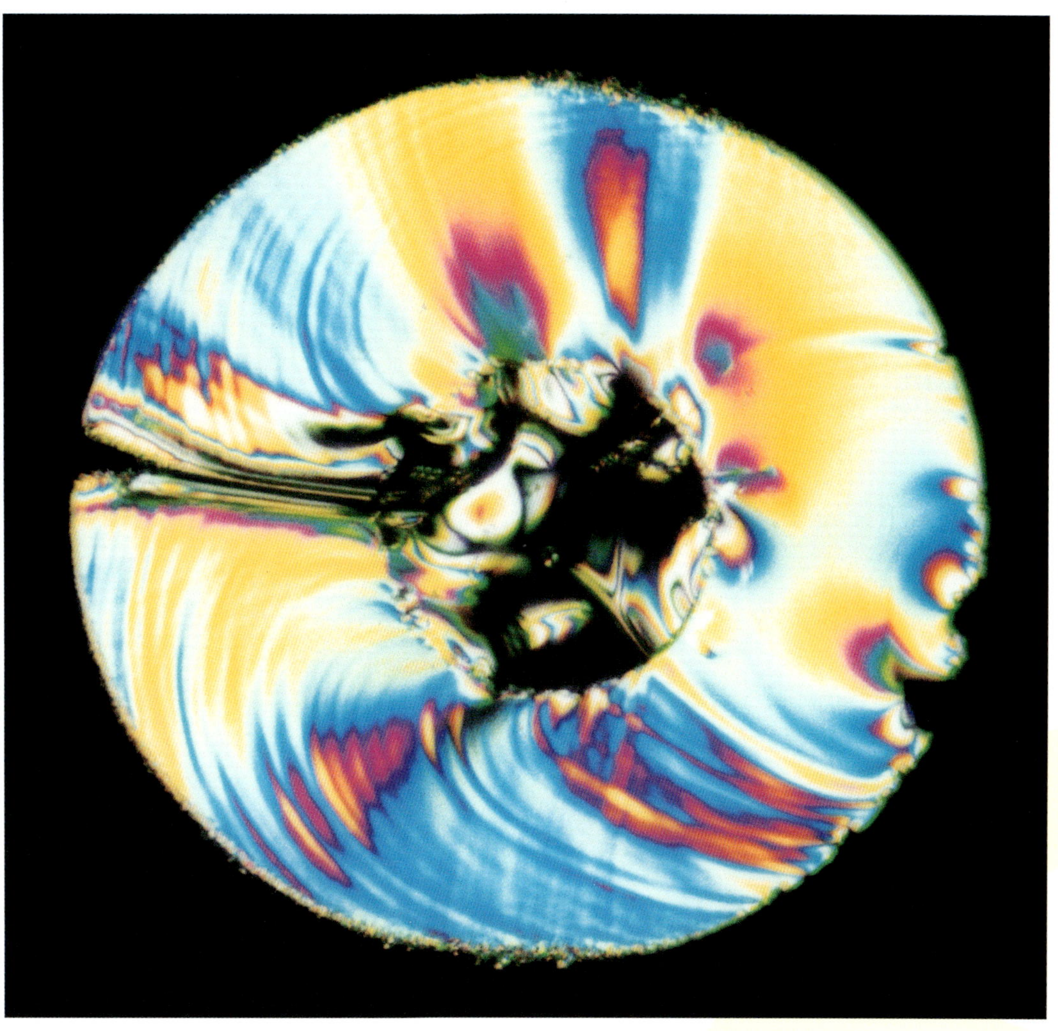

Materials property design of fiber-reinforced ceramic matrix composites

The mechanical performance of fiber-reinforced ceramic matrix composites has been analyzed using properties of fiber, matrix, and interface. The theoretical predictions are compared with simple model materials. The photograph shows a typical example of the fracture surface of glass fiber-reinforced glass matrix monofilament composite. The effect of elastic modulus and thermal expansion coefficient of the fiber and matrix on tensile fracture behavior has been compared with theoretical analysis.

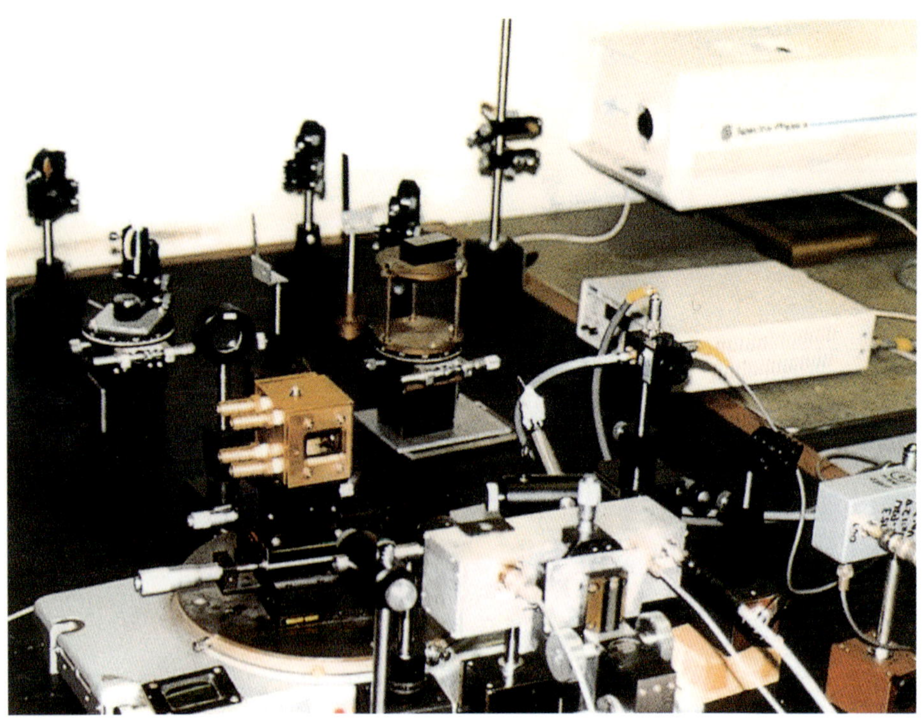

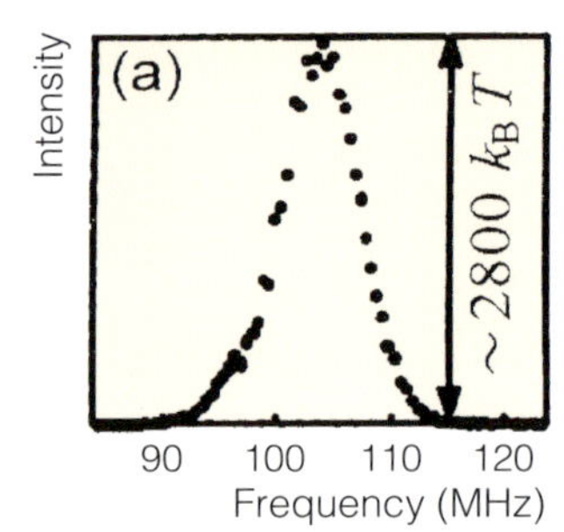

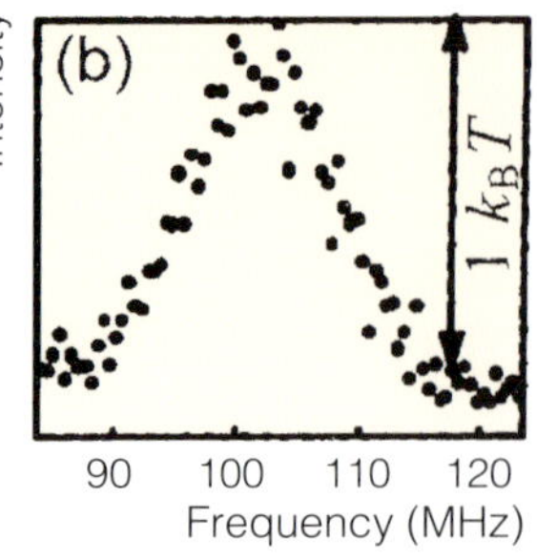

Wide-band phnon generation by an amplitude modulated laser

A coherent phonon was generated in liquid by a laser. The laser illuminates a thin metal film formed on a flat surface of a sapphire rod immersed in a sample liquid. The intensity of the induced phonon is flat over a wide frequency range. The excited phonon (fig. (a)) has an intensity 2800 times that of the spontaneous phonon (fig. (b)).

3-D segmented optical waveguides

A light beam propagates in a waveguide because light is confined in high refractive-index regions. We fabricated a new type of waveguide, which consists of the segmented high index regions, in a litium niobate crystal. This waveguide can be fabricated with high-density and flexible structures, such as a curve or a branch. The picture shows the output pattern of a Y-branched waveguide.

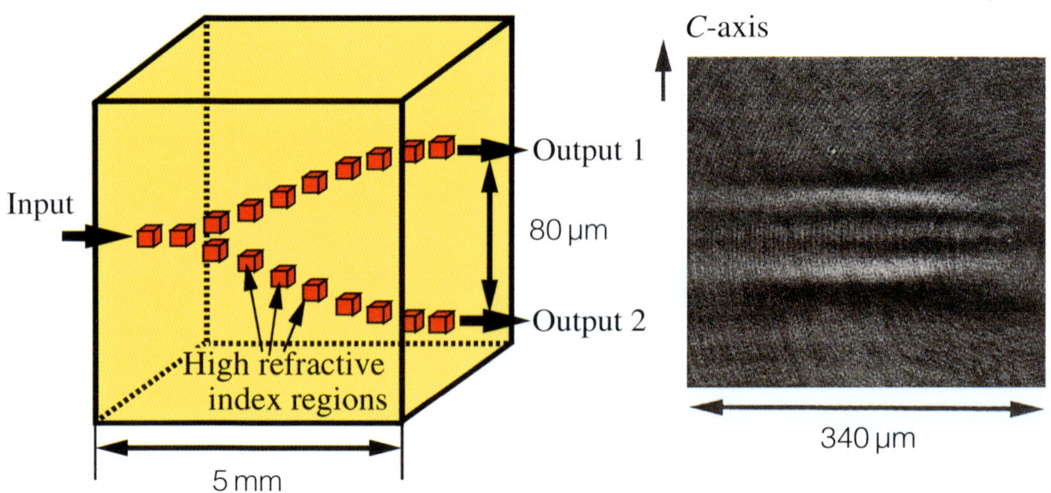

Improvement of the beam quality of high power laser diode

High power laser diodes have the problem of a poor beam quality, that is a wide spectrum and a wide diverging angle. We improved these by the technique of injection locking. By injecting a high quality beam from another laser into the active layer, we obtained a high power and high quality laser beam, which is quite useful for various applications.

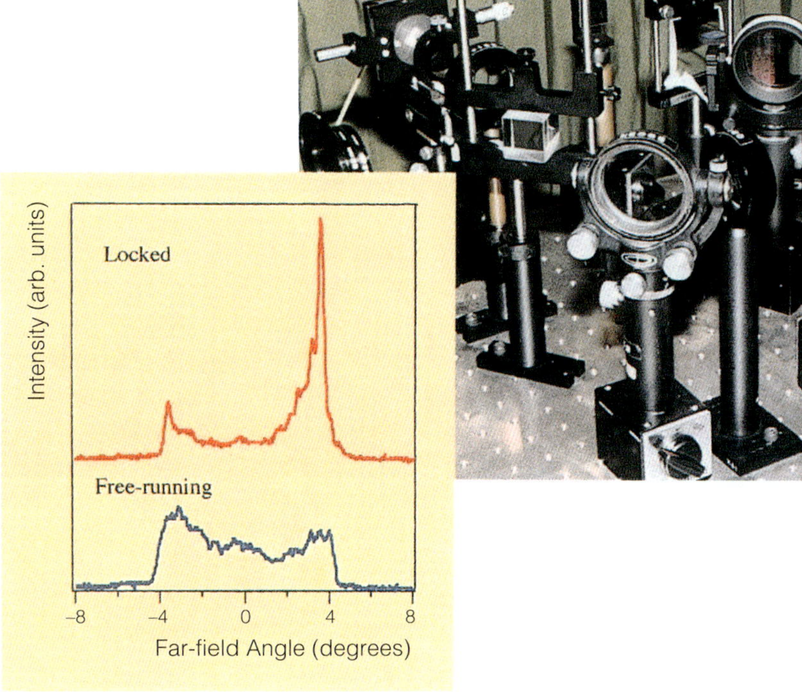

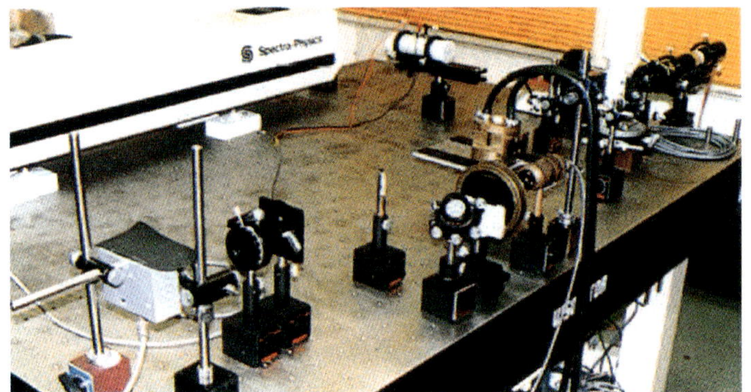

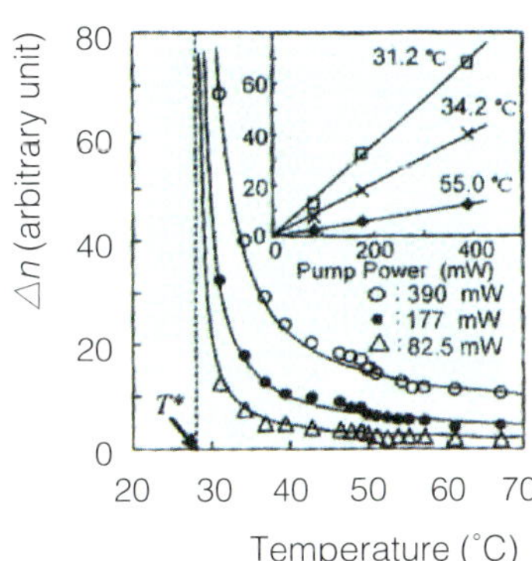

Local molecular orientational order induced by CW laser

While rod-like molecules are randomly oriented in a liquid phase, we can put their orientation in order by using a laser beam. Induced birefringence Δn, which represents the degree of the orientational order, increases when the laser power is increased or the temperature of the liquid approaches the critical level.

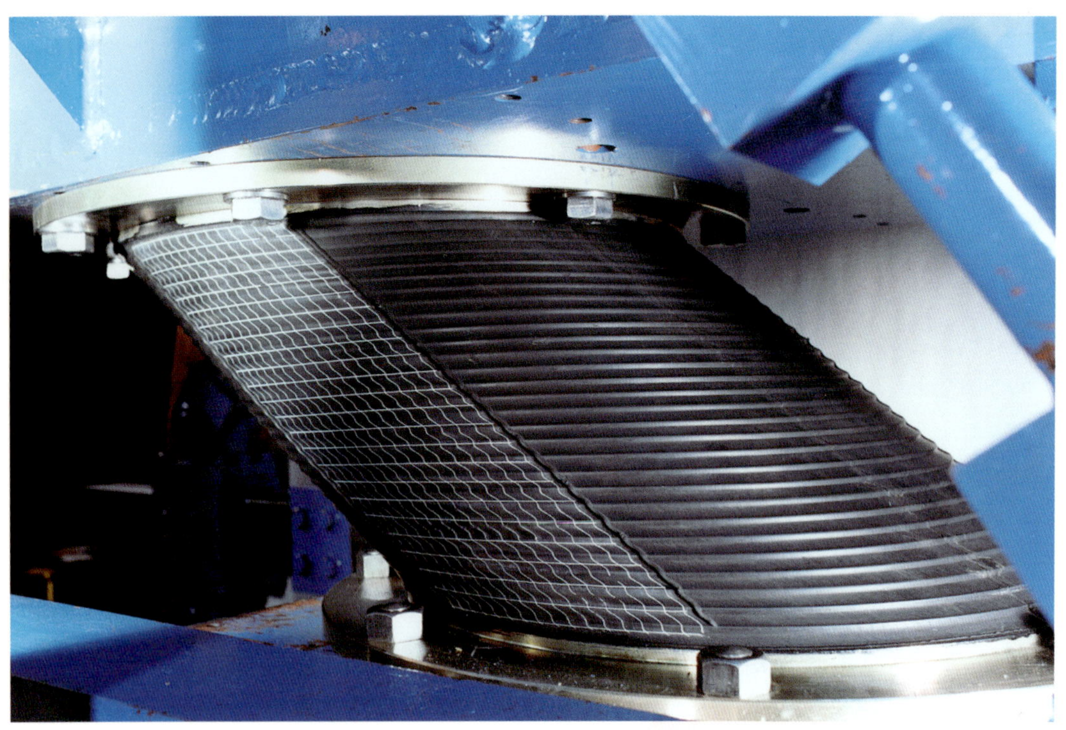

Seismic isolation technology to attenuate vibrations of buildings caused by earthquakes

Seismic isolation of buildings owes its present applications to development of reliable laminated rubber bearings, which are used to support the buildings. The figure shows that a rubber bearing comprising 30 rubber sheets of 440 mm diameter and 5 mm thickness bonded to steel plates of 3 mm thickness, could be stable under conditions of a 1960 kN vertical load and a 300 mm displacement (about 3/4 times the diameter).

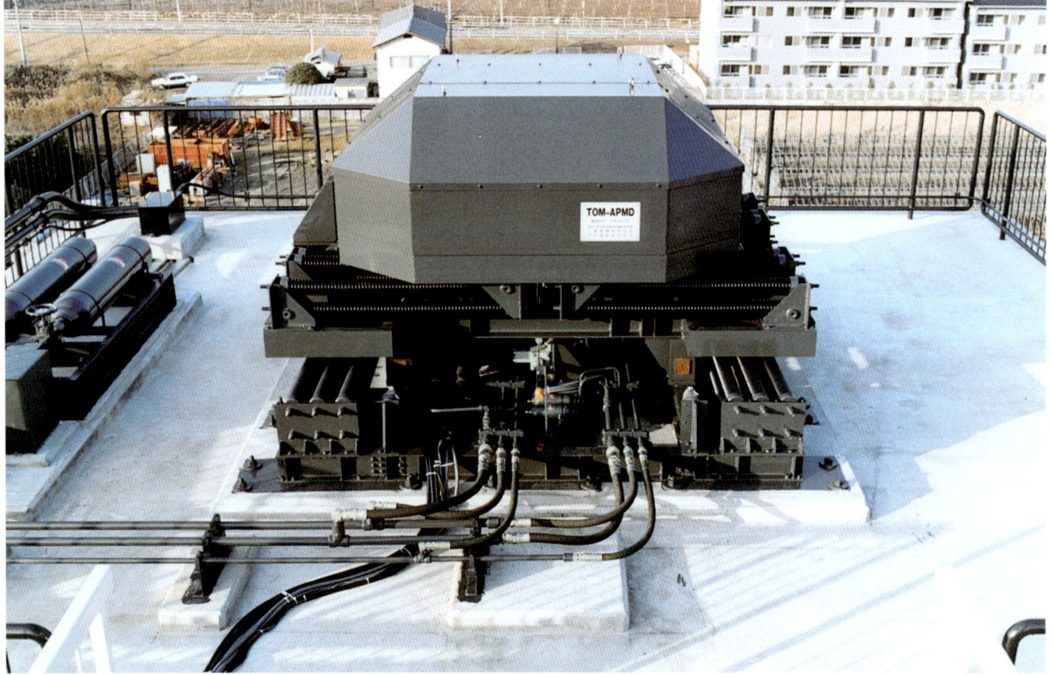

Active vibration control technology to attenuate vibrations of buildings induced by strong winds

For control of wind-induced vibrations in tall buildings, mass dampers with moving masses of 1/200 to 1/100 times the total mass of the buildings are installed on the roofs or the top floors of the buildings, in order to make reaction forces produced by the moving masses act as damping forces for the buildings. Particularly active mass dampers can achieve high performance vibration control by controlling the motion of the moving masses in accordance with vibration states of the buildings. The figure shows a large-scale experimental model of an active mass damper using hydraulic actuators.

If the movement can be accurately controlled, it might be useful in improving comfort in a vehicle, suppressing the shaking of buildings, or machining brittle materials with no cracks. The combination between the mechanism and the control technology is very important.

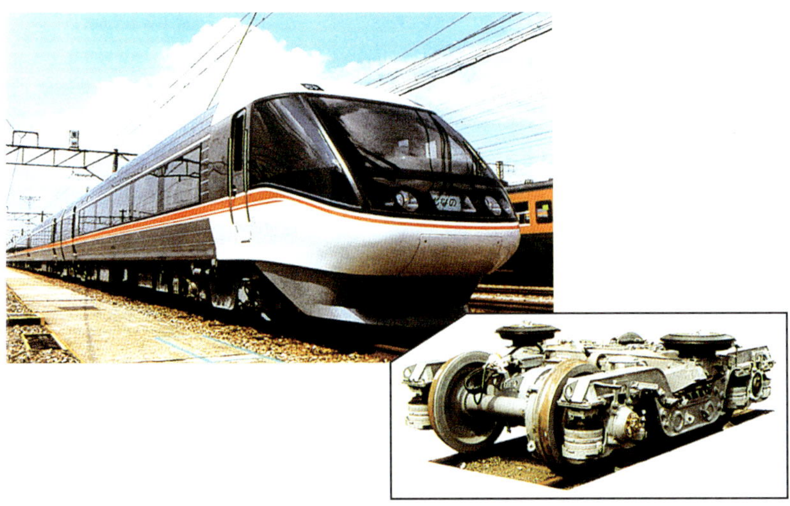

Self-steering railway truck with asymmetrical suspension

The improvement of curving performance for railway vehicles on curved track on Japanese conventional lines is important. The concept of asymmetrical fore-and-aft suspension was proposed for a self-steering truck, and was introduced in the fastest pendulum train "Wide View Shinano" for curve negotiation in Japan. A reduction of wear between wheel and rail can be achieved. The stiffness of the truck suspension is switched by a pneumatic actuator according to the direction of travel.

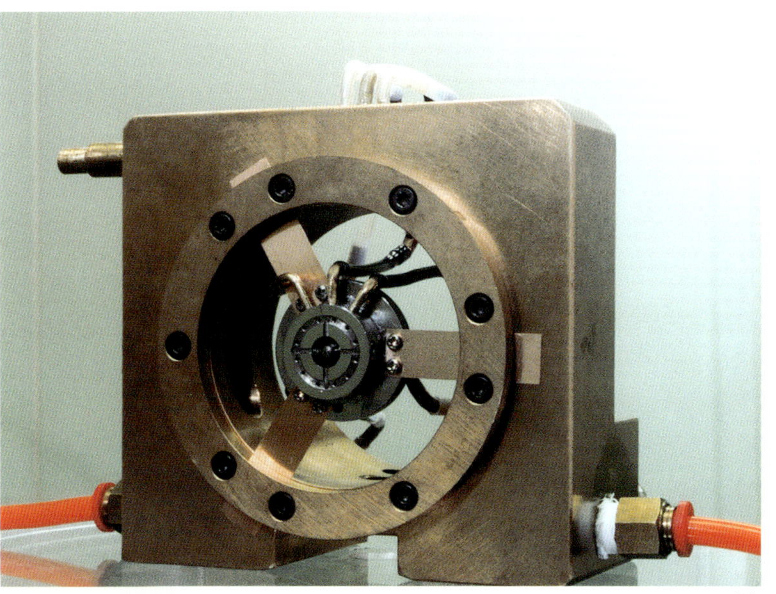

(a)

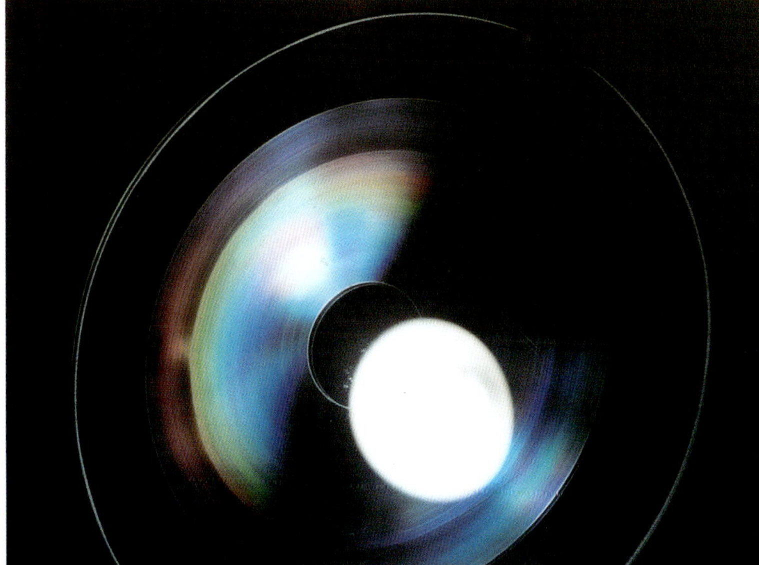

(b)

Ductile regime cutting of optical glass using a negative-pressure flying tool

It is necessary to cut to a very small depth of less than 0.1 μm in order to machine glass with no cracks. However any accurate machine tool has error motions and vibrations of the same value. So a negative-pressure flying tool was developed to cut mirror surfaces, because the system kept a constant distance between the tool and the workpiece using the action of vacuum suction.

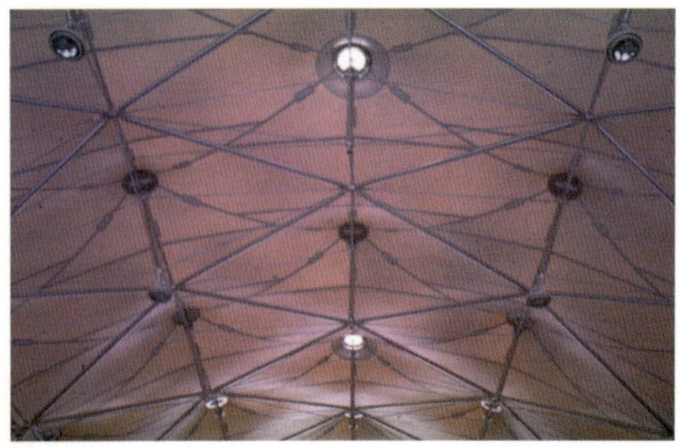

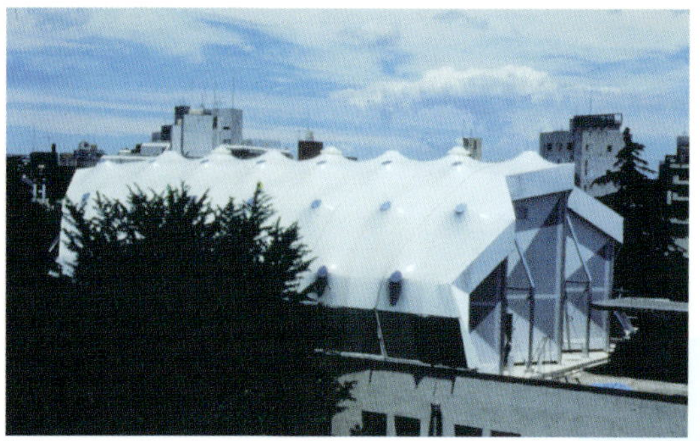

The development of large space structures

One of the main objectives in the design of large space structures is to develop lightweight structures. Truss structures stabilized by a cable tension system, as shown in the photos, have been developed as one of the lightest steel structures. This dome structure is used for research not only for structural engineering but also for air conditioning and acoustics.

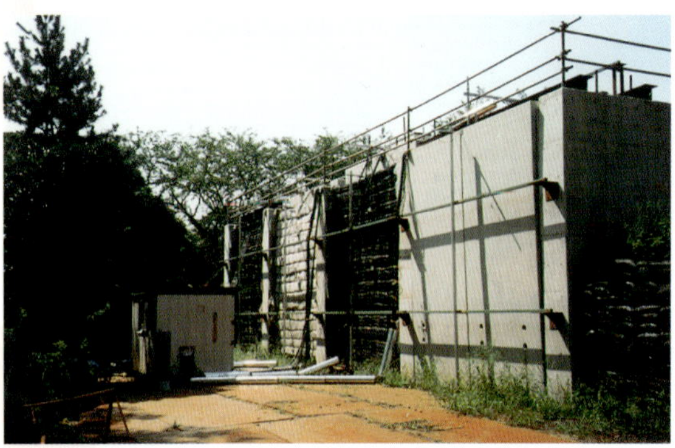

Development of reinforced soil retaining walls

Reinforced soil retaining walls consist of backfill soils reinforced by synthetic grids or textiles and very thin concrete facing walls. They can reduce the total cost of construction while increasing the stability of structures. Above all, good seismic performance was obtained during the 1995 Hanshin-Awazi earthquake disaster. Currently, full-scale model tests are performed to further increase their stability.

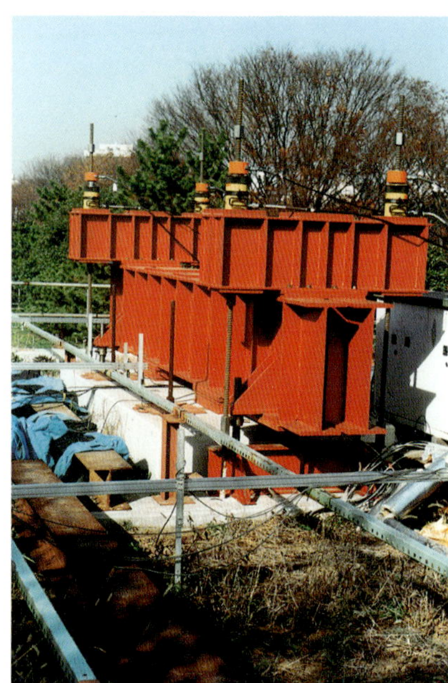
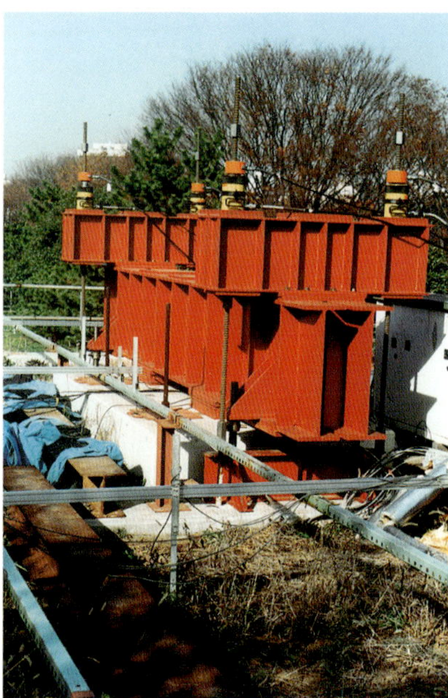

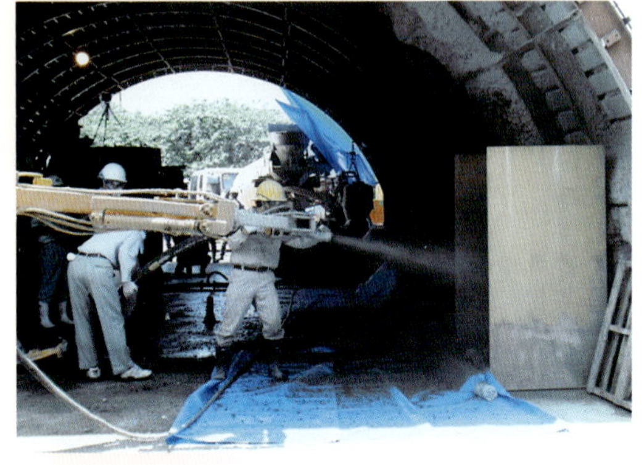
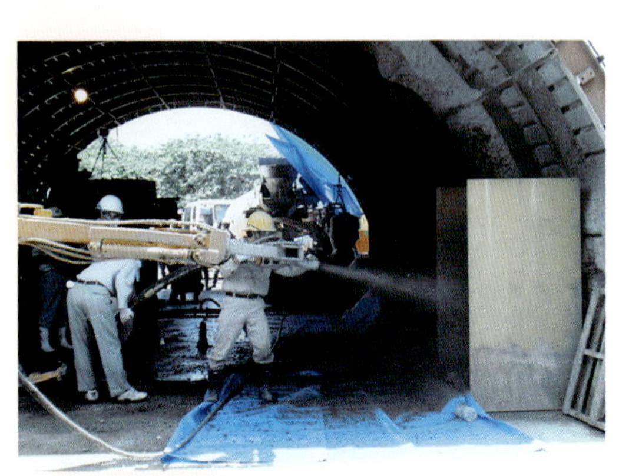

Development of high quality shotcrete

Shotcrete has been widely using in tunnel and underground projects, in surface protection, preparation and reinforcement of concrete structures. At this time, it is essential that detailed specifications of the construction method as well as the quality of shotcrete are recorded. A high quality shotcrete is under development based on analysis (DEM model) and experiments from a tunnel model.

Substructure On-Line Pseudo-dynamic testing of a 2-bay, 12-story R/C building

The Substructure On-Line Pseudo-dynamic test consists of a numerical analysis and loading test, in which a member or subassemblage of an entire structure is loaded and the measured hysteretic characteristics are incorporated in the analysis while others are numerically assumed. One of the advantages of this technique compared with a shaking table test is that the seismic characteristics of large-scale or high-rise buildings can be studied more easily.

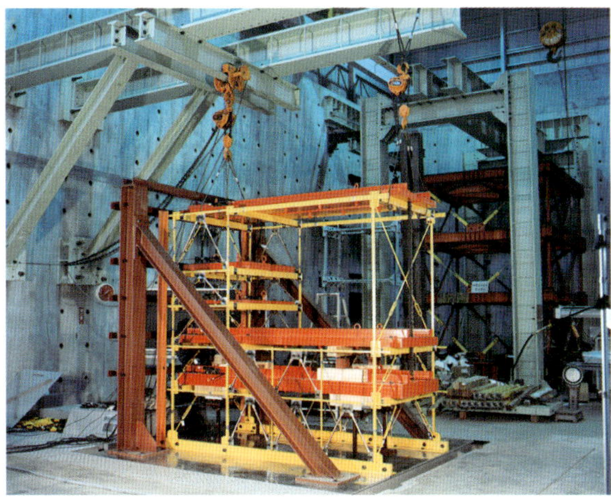

Shaking table test on a scaled model of industrial building

Most industrial buildings have complicated features of frame which are different from those of ordinary office buildings. These features are directly reflected into difficulties in seismic design. In order to investigate the inelastic earthquake responses of these types of buildings, a scaled model of a three-story electric power plant building was tested on the shaking table.

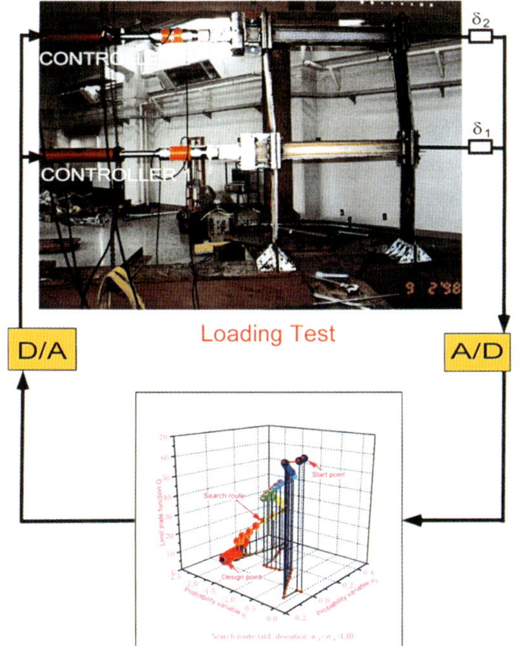

Hybrid search for design points combined with computer-controlled loading tests

This figure shows a block diagram of a hybrid testing system, where a design point searching process in the reliability analysis is combined with computer-controlled loading tests. A deterministic structural model subjected to uncertain load profile is driven to the most likely failure situation by this system.

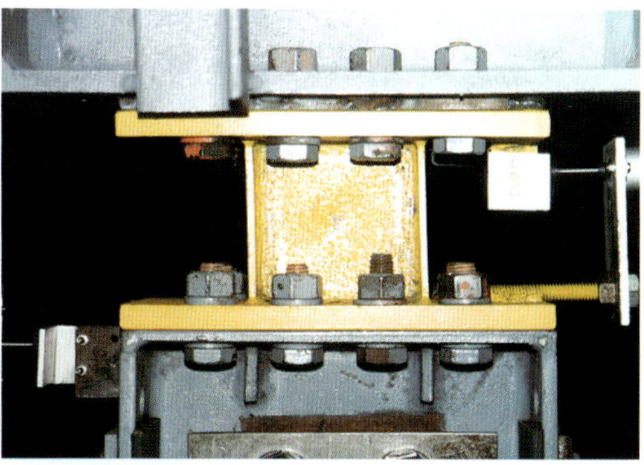

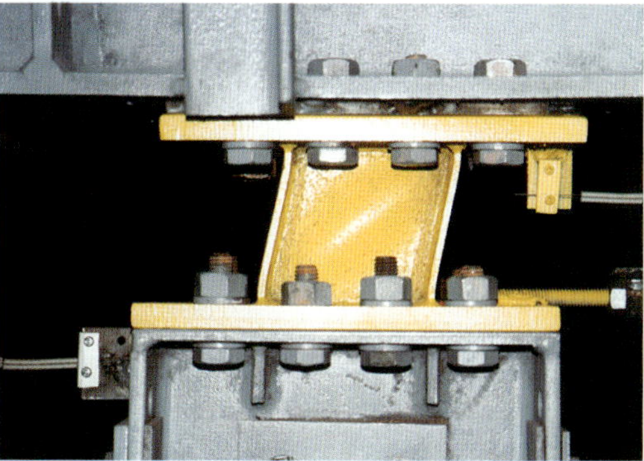

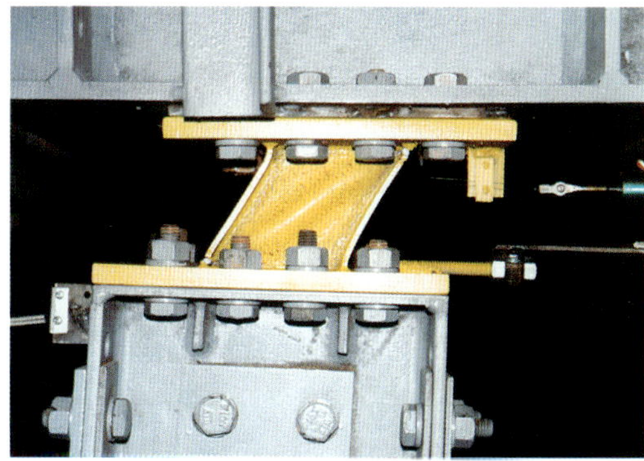

Pseudo-dynamic tests on a steel frame with hysteretic dampers

Hysteretic dampers made of low-yield-point steel are expected to reduce the response of structures not only in designing new buildings but also in retrofitting existing buildings. To study the non-linear earthquake responses of the whole structure model, substructuring pseudo-dynamic tests are carried out.

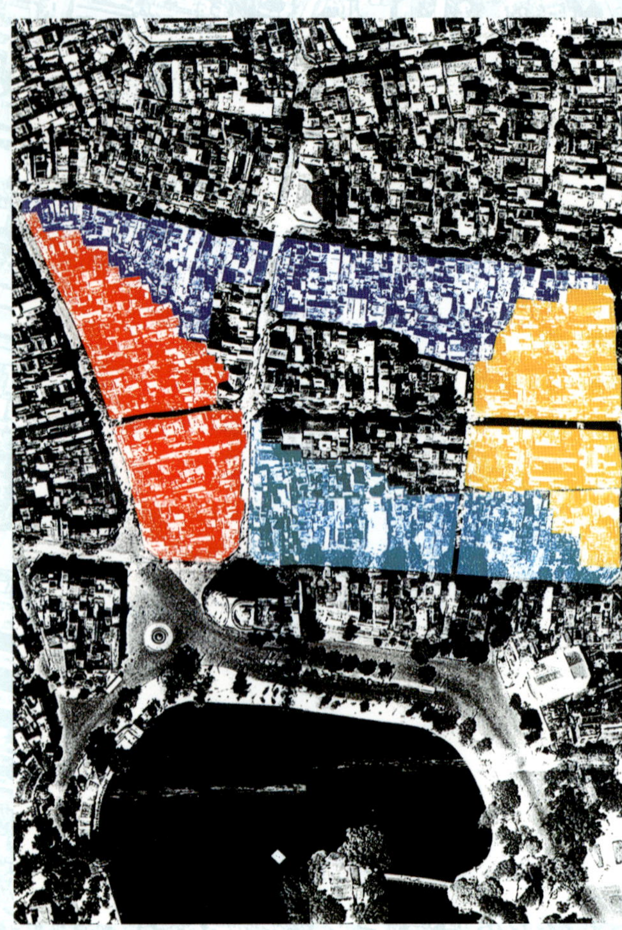

Block composition of Hanoi, Vietnam

The block composition of Hanoi, Vietnam, reflects the long history of the city. There is a district called "36 Street District" in the middle of the old city, where extremely long and narrow houses such as 2.5 m × 60 m can be seen. Although the space composition looks strange, some common mechanisms of the local life, the climate and the history can be seen in it. The figure shows the process of how the district has been filled up, and how the streets were planned to run through there.

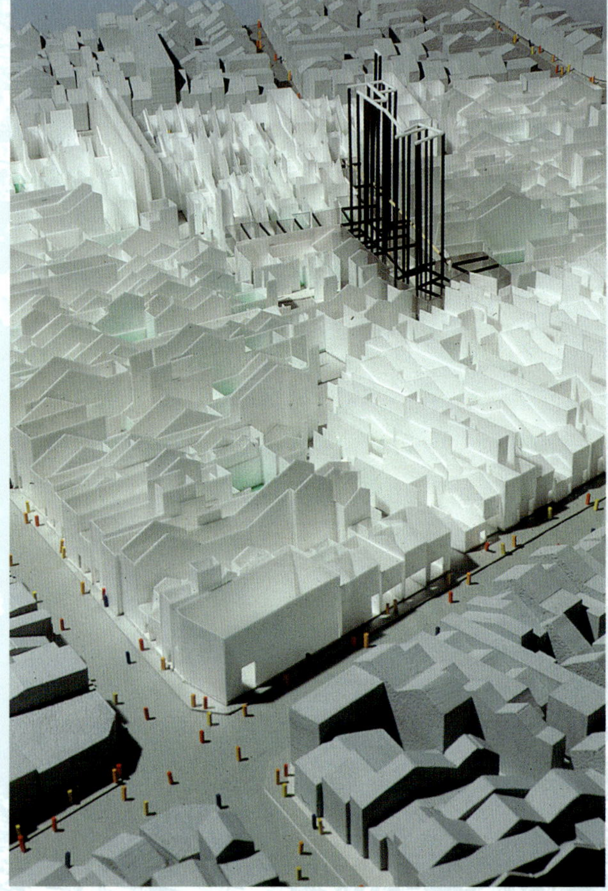

The model of a dense residential city block in Hanoi, Vietnam

In the modern universal urban planning, it is considered important that the urban space composition should have gradual scales and gradual functions. However, there are only two elements in the space composition of the "36 Street District", the "midtown street" and the "completely private street". The figure shows a virtual model of a residential block where the "intermediate scale of space" is introduced. Insertion of a new element brings a new mutual relationship. This may lead to the birth of a new town in this place.

Since everyone is the "hero" of their own "way of life," its hard for anyone to be objective about "living." Cities, where 'living' is gathered together en masse, are at once convenient and distant. We must therefore make every effort to understand what cities actually are.

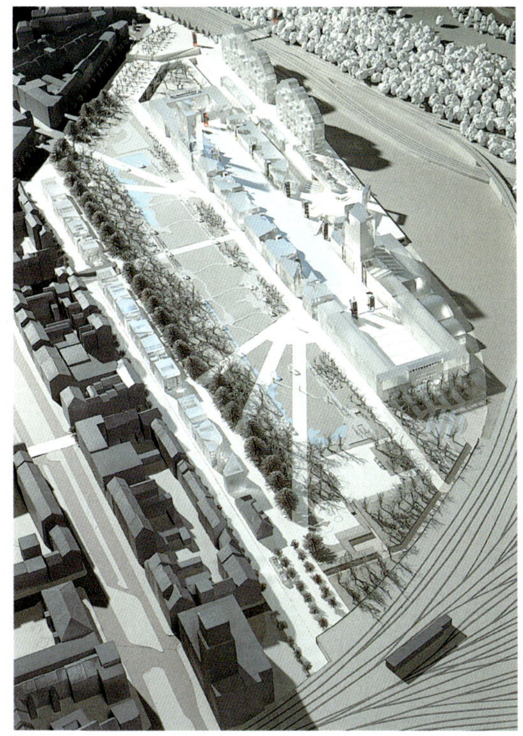

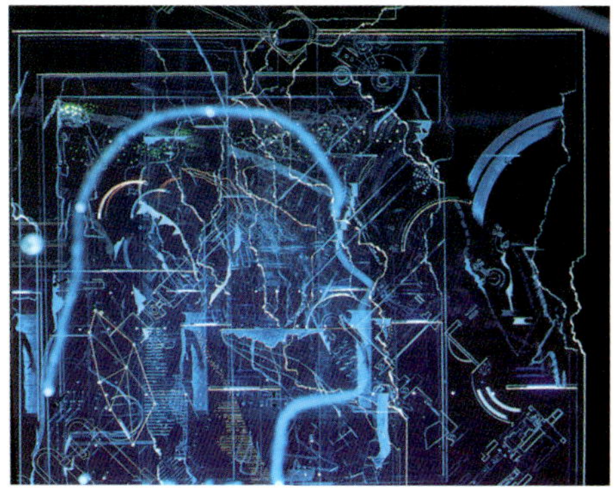

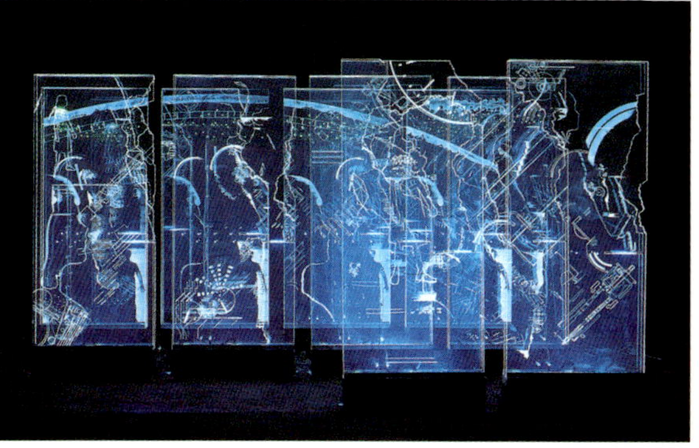

Modal space of consciousness-shadow robot

This is a work shown in the exhibition held in Minneapolis, USA. Visitors can walk among these objects. In the exhibition space, there stood acrylic panels with several kinds of electric lights. They were programmed to be an orchestra playing "music by light." Light and darkness are delicately programmed and gave silent pulse to the space, like the ebb and flow of the tide. What "form" can change our perception and the space? This is a kind of experimental device.

Proposal for media park, Köln

Architectural design competitions ask for both clearness in logical concepts of space, and the skill to give them concrete form. Not only one but many "right answers" are produced for a given subject, but the problem of spatial evaluation cannot have an absolute index, and the answers can be found in applied proposals. In this design competition, the main subject was "expression of the contemporary center of information by architecture". Our answer to this question tries to find the intrinsic essence of communication in a sender and a receiver, in a "human" sense.

(500 m × 500 m × 500 m) cube for a hundred thousand residents

A real world city shows so many functions and variation of processes. There are a hundred stories in a hundred cities, and if we look into the future, there are infinitely many possibilities also. It is difficult to obtain the knowledge of how to create a new generation city by only studying how a real city is now. The figure is a piece of drawing from a series of works that tried to show the process of a virtual city. It is an imaginary description of "a general history of urban space", of layered order and disorder, and a burst of new forms.

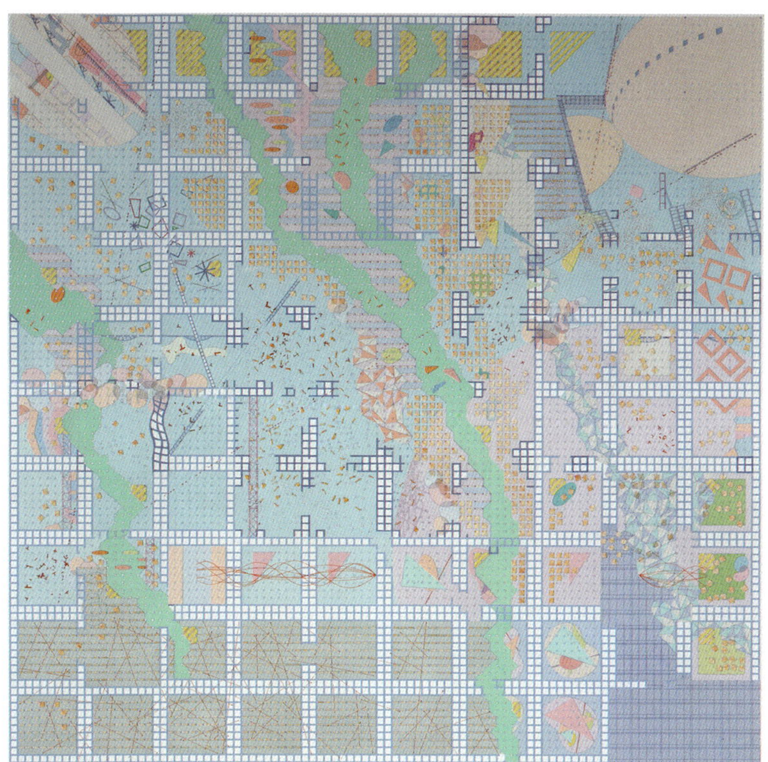

The study field of engineering is one that has very close links to society as a whole. Engineering research to date has enriched the lives of persons around the globe, but it has also greatly endangered the lives of many people of this generation and of generations to come.

Let us imagine for a moment a world of science whose objective was purely and simply the acquisition of knowledge.

In such a world, research must begin with the rather gloomy assumption that truth already exists a priori in the systems of nature. We can only test approaches to understanding the already-existing nature of those systems.

In engineering, on the other hand, it is essential that the motivation to make things be the desire to meet the wants and needs of people. And those wants and needs cannot be fully understood unless we assume that society is made up of people who are consumed by desire and that many contradictions are enveloped within that desire. Unless one is able to comprehend the emotions of wanting something that has added convenience or something that is easier to use, one cannot really understand the essence of engineering. And this requires one to search for that separate 'something' that comprises truth in nature.

Let us imagine, as an example, we are climbing an as-yet unexplored mountain, one that has but a single peak. We have just left the foot of the mountain, which is shrouded in mist so that we cannot well see where we are going. The mountain has only one peak, so our strategy is simply to climb and climb until we cannot climb any higher. There are any number of routes going up to the top, and since they all lead to the peak all of them could be called the 'right road'.

Now let us imagine the mist-shrouded mountain is one that has multiple peaks, a fact of which we are unaware. We scale and conquer dizzying precipices again and again, and finally (we think) reach the summit. And just then the mist suddenly clears up, and we see there is another, higher peak far in the distance. All that work for nothing! We were wrong from the very first step! We took the wrong road!

Well, we'll just have to make the best of it. It's lucky in a way; if the mist hadn't cleared up we would never have realized that we climbed the wrong peak. But maybe the road we took has been closed due to snow. People coming after us may have to take a different route. Maybe the peak is on a different part of land, separated by a deep sea so that no one can climb it.

Maybe, after all, it would have been better if the mist hadn't cleared up. Then we would have been satisfied that we had gotten up to here.

Whether we like it or not, it is of processes like this that today's society is made up. In some cases, people make things that afterward are used in ways the maker could not have imagined. Alfred Nobel's inventing of dynamite springs to mind as an example. There are countless examples we can recall of things that were initially made with the noblest of intentions, but that only a short time later brought misfortune and misery to mankind. Witness weapons and wars, symbolized by the development of atomic bombs; traffic accidents; the destruction of the environment by pollution, deforestation and the like; global warming; depletion of natural resources; the population boom......

It may well be that the 'new engineering' now being sought will be characterized by the question, "How can we NOT make things?"

On the other hand, though, people will certainly continue to treasure the sheer joy of creating new things. That is why we continue to make things. I earnestly hope readers will, as they encounter the advanced research developments that appear throughout the text, try to visualize the research sites where these developments were made. There are a great many people at these sites who bring a real sense of joy to their work. They know the pain of failure and the sweat of hard toil, but they also know the joy of creation, of putting all their energies into making things to satisfy the desires of many. The research developments presented in this book are all embodiments of the application of those energies.

To give the reader a bit of background information on Institute of Industrial Science, University of Tokyo (I.I.S.), the research institute that figures prominently in this book, it was converted in 1949 from what had been the University of Tokyo's 2nd Engineering School. In the first 10 years of its existence it was located on the Chiba campus, and in 1962 shifted from its war-era status as a living quarters for the 7th infantry division of the Imperial army to a full-fledged scientific organization dedicated to the cause of peace.

The Institute's existence as a breeding ground for engineers needed for WWII ended with the end of that war. It is ironic that the campus location eventually was shifted to Roppongi, a place which holds many wartime memories for Japanese, and in a way the conversion to its peacetime role symbolizes that of Japan as a whole.

In any event, the result of this shift was that the Institute was ultimately located in the center of the thriving, bustling metropolis of Tokyo, from where it could change to keep pace with the dynamic changes in industry and society occurring around it. This greatly influenced the manner in which the lab conducted its activities after that.

In 1999, I.I.S. is celebrating the 50th anniversary of its founding in Tokyo's Meguro Ward, a move that reflects the restructuring of the University of Tokyo as a whole to meet societal changes that have occurred around it. In its new location, I.I.S. will continue to fulfill its role in society as part of the University of Tokyo, along with the university's other campuses in central Tokyo and in Kashiwa. No other research organization, from its founding up until the present time, can be said to more accurately reflect the industry and society of which it is a part.

*　*　*

I have already referred to the joy that comes with creating things, but would like to emphasize once again the enjoyment that this joy brings to our work as researchers. It is precisely for this reason that we must continue to strive for further successes. I trust that the readers of this book will, as fellow travelers on the journey of life in which we all participate, bear with us as we continue this endeavor.

reference

substance

p.12 ·········· Suzuki, T. Lab., Edagawa, K.,Lab.
p.13 ·········· Okano, T. Lab., Fukutani, K. Lab.
p.14 ·········· top : Mitsuda, Y. Lab., bottom : Mori, M. Lab.
p.15 ·········· top, bottom : Nihei, Y. Lab.
p.16 ·········· Nihei, Y. Lab.
p.17 ·········· top : Mori, M. Lab., Ishida, Y. Lab., bottom : Mizobe, Y. Lab.
p.18 ·········· top : Fasol, G. Lab., middle, bottom : Sakaki, H. Lab.
p.19 ·········· top, middle, bottom : Arakawa, Y. Lab.
p.20 ·········· top, bottom : Kagawa, Y. Lab.
p.21 ·········· top, bottom left / right : Kagawa, Y. Lab.
p.22 ·········· top, bottom : Masuzawa, T. Lab.
p.23 ·········· top : Nakagawa, T. Lab., bottom : Tani, Y. Lab.
p.24 ·········· top, bottom : Fujita, H. Lab.
p.25 ·········· top, bottom : Fujita, H. Lab.
p.26 ·········· top, bottom : Watanabe, T. Lab.
p.27 ·········· Nihei, Y. Lab.
p.28 ·········· top : Yasui, I. Lab., bottom : Sakoda, A. Lab.
p.29 ·········· top, bottom : Yamamoto, R. Lab.
p.30 ·········· top : Tokunaga, M. Lab., middle, bottom : Musiake, K. Lab.
p.31 ·········· top : Yamazaki, F. Lab., bottom : Meguro, K. Lab.
p.32 ·········· top : Yasuoka, Y. Lab., Shibasaki, R. Lab., bottom : Murai, S. Lab., Shibasaki, R. Lab.
p.33 ·········· top, bottom : Oki, T. Lab.
p.34 ·········· top : Murai, S. Lab., Shibasaki, R. Lab., bottom : Suzuki, M. Lab., Sakoda, A. Lab.
p.35 ·········· Murai, S. Lab., Shibasaki, R. Lab.

phenomenon

p.38 ·········· top : Kobayashi, T. Lab., bottom : Nishio, S. Lab.
p.39 ·········· top : Kobayashi, T. Lab., Taniguchi, N. Lab., bottom : Kobayashi, T. Lab.
p.40 ·········· Yokoi, H. Lab.
p.41 ·········· top : Kimura, Y. Lab., bottom left : Kawakatsu, H. Lab., bottom right : Kimura, Y. Lab.
p.42 ·········· top : Yokoi, H. Lab., bottom : Nakagawa, T. Lab.
p.43 ·········· Nishio, S. Lab.
p.44 ·········· top, bottom : Murakami, S. Lab., Kato, S. Lab.

p.45 ·········· top, bottom : Murakami, S. Lab., Kato, S. Lab.
p.46 ·········· top : Ishii, M. Lab., middle : Hirakawa, K. Lab., bottom : Ishii, M. Lab.
p.47 ·········· top : Hirakawa, K. Lab., middle : Fujii, Y. Lab., bottom : Ishii, M. Lab.
p.48 ·········· Kuroda, K. Lab., Shimura, T. Lab.
p.49 ·········· Takagi, K. Lab., Sakai, K. Lab.
p.50 ·········· top : Tachibana, H. Lab., Tokyu Construction CO.,LTD., bottom : Tachibana, H. Lab.
p.51 ·········· top, bottom : Tachibana, H. Lab.

discovery

p.66 ·········· top : Tanaka, H. Lab., bottom : Konagai, K. Lab.
p.67 ·········· top : Konagai, K. Lab., bottom : Tanaka, H. Lab.
p.68 ·········· Watanabe, K. Lab.
p.69 ·········· top, bottom : Watanabe, K. Lab.
p.70 ·········· top, bottom : Yoshikawa, N. Lab.
p.71 ·········· top : Hangai, Y. Lab., Kawaguchi, K. Lab., bottom : Nakagiri, S. Lab.
p.72 ·········· Yoshiki, H. Lab.
p.73 ·········· top : Nishio, S. Lab., bottom : Yanagimoto, J. Lab.
p.74 ·········· top, bottom : Hangai, Y. Lab., Kawaguchi, K. Lab.
p.75 ·········· Hangai, Y. Lab., Kawaguchi, K. Lab.
p.76 ·········· top, bottom : Toi, Y. Lab.
p.77 ·········· top, bottom : Toi, Y. Lab.
p.78 ·········· top : Kobayashi, T. Lab., Taniguchi, N. Lab., bottom : Oshima, M. Lab., Taniguchi, N. Lab., Kobayashi, T. Lab.
p.79 ·········· top, bottom : Kobayashi, T. Lab., Taniguchi, N. Lab.
p.80 ·········· top : Suzuki, M. Lab., Sakai, Y. Lab., bottom : Suzuki, M. Lab., Sakoda, A. Lab.
p.81 ·········· Uryu, T. Lab.
p.82 ·········· top : Sezaki, K. Lab., bottom : Sato, Y. Lab.
p.83 ·········· top : Ikeuchi, K. Lab., Sato, Y. Lab., middle, bottom : Ikeuchi, K. Lab.
p.84 ·········· top, bottom : Sakauchi, M. Lab.
p.85 ·········· top left : Takaba, S. Lab., top right : Tatemura, J. Lab., bottom left : Yasuda, Y. Lab., bottom right : Imai, H. Lab.
p.86 ·········· Kuwahara, M. Lab.
p.87 ·········· top : Meguro, K. Lab., bottom : Kuwahara, M. Lab.
p.88 ·········· top, bottom : Yamazaki, F. Lab.

p.89 ·········· top : International Center for Disaster-Mitigation Engineering, University of Tokyo, middle : Herath, A.S. Lab., bottom : Meguro, K. Lab.

invention

p.92 ·········· top : Ura, T. Lab., bottom : Maeda, H. Lab., Courtesy of Mega-Float Technical Research Association
p.93 ·········· top : Ura, T. Lab., bottom : Maeda, H. Lab.
p.94 ·········· top : Harashima, F. Lab., Hashimoto, H. Lab., bottom : Hashimoto, H. Lab.
p.95 ·········· top : Harashima, F. Lab., Hashimoto, H. Lab., bottom left / right : Hashimoto, H. Lab.
p.96 ·········· Fujita, H. Lab.
p.97 ·········· top left, top right, bottom : Fujita, H. Lab.
p.98 ·········· top : Kitsuregawa, M. Lab., middle : Sakaki, H. Lab., Hirakawa, K. Lab., bottom : Hirakawa, K. Lab.
p.99 ·········· top left : Hiramoto, T. Lab., top right : Sakurai, T. Lab., bottom : Toshiyoshi, H. Lab.
p.100 ········ top : Okano, T. Lab., Fukutani, K. Lab., bottom : Suzuki, T. Lab., Edagawa, K.,Lab.
p.101 ········ Maeda, H. Lab.
p.102 ········ top : Sakaki, H. Lab., Arakawa, Y. Lab., bottom left : Hiramoto, T. Lab., bottom right : Arakawa, Y. Lab.
p.103 ········ top, bottom : Arakawa, Y. Lab.
p.104 ········ Kato, T. Lab.
p.105 ········ top, bottom : Araki, K. Lab.
p.106 ········ top : Nanao, S. Lab., bottom : Kudo, T. Lab.
p.107 ········ Kagawa, Y. Lab.
p.110 ········ top, bottom : Fujita, T. Lab.
p.111 ········ left : Suda, Y. Lab., right : Tani, Y. Lab.
p.112 ········ top : Hangai, Y. Lab., Kawaguchi, K. Lab., Fujii, A. Lab., middle left : Koseki, J. Lab., middle right : Nakano, Y. Lab., bottom : Uomoto, K. Lab.
p.113 ········ top left, bottom left, right : Ohi, K. Lab.
p.114 ········ left, background photo : Fujimori, T. Lab., Magaribuchi, H. Lab., right : Magaribuchi, H. Lab.
p.115 ········ top left, top right, bottom : Hara, H. Lab., Fujii, A. Lab., Magaribuchi, H. Lab.

index

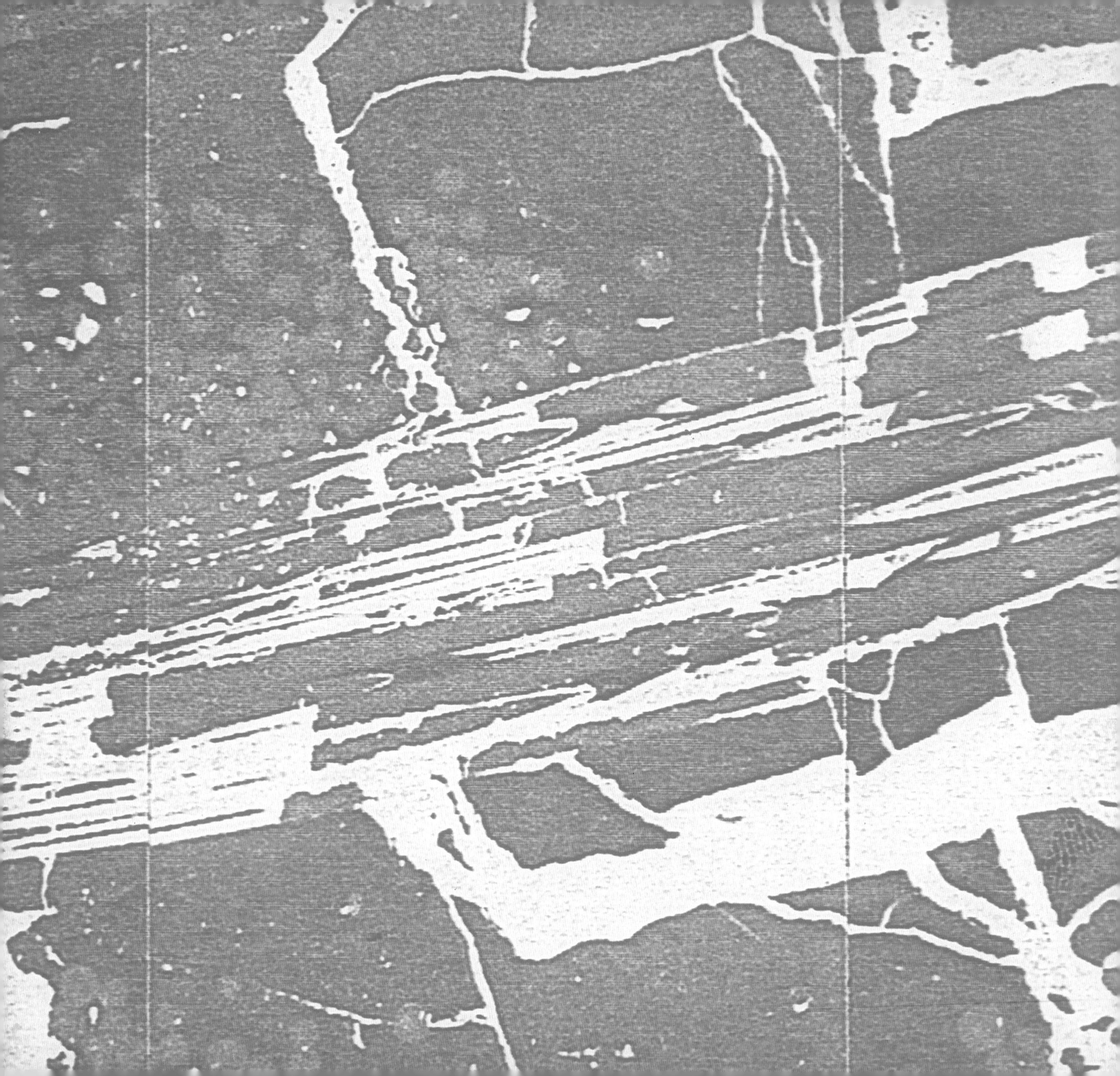